Evaluation and Treatment of Swallowing Disorders

Evaluation and Treatment of Swallowing Disorders

by
Jeri A. Logemann, PhD
Chairman, Communicative Disorders
The School of Speech
Northwestern University
Evanston, Illinois

College-Hill Press, Inc., San Diego, CA

College-Hill Press, Inc.
4284 41st Street
San Diego, California 92105

Library of Congress Cataloging in Publication Data

Logemann, Jerilyn A., date-
  Evaluation and treatment of swallowing disorders.

  Bibliography: p.
  Includes index.
  1. Deglutition disorders. I. Title. [DNLM:
1. Deglutition disorders. 2. Deglutition disorders—
Rehabilitation. WI 250 L832e]
RC815.2.L63 1983   616.3'1   83-7234
ISBN 0-933014-84-8

Printed in the United States of America

Contents

Author Index   238

Subject Index

Preface

This volume is intended to present the current state of the art in research and clinical management of patients with difficulty in feeding orally, particularly those who are aspirating. It is an attempt to coalesce the various literatures in medical and allied health journals and publications devoted to management of dysphagia, with the author's 10 years of research in the area. Normal physiology of deglutition is reviewed and techniques for the evaluation and treatment of dysphagia are detailed. Methodologies advocated reflect the author's prejudices for a conservative approach including detailed radiographic evaluation of swallowing dysfunction in conjunction with careful clinical examination. This book emphasizes the use of data from these detailed diagnostic batteries in the development of therapy/management programs. This conservative philosophy is based on the author's perceived need for procedures to handle dysphagia that are relatively safe medically and that, therefore, put the patient, physician, and swallowing therapist (whichever professional may be playing this role) at minimal risk.

The issue of which professional should assume the role of swallowing therapist has not been addressed in detail. Currently, no profession is consistently educating its members in the diagnosis and treatment of dysphagia. However, speech and language pathology training programs are beginning to incorporate courses in dysphagia in their curriculums. The speech pathologist has extensive experience in feeding programs, particularly with cerebral palsy patients, and has background information on head and neck anatomy. However, without sufficient coursework and experience in diagnosis and management of a wide variety of dysphagic patients, a speech pathologist or other professional may fail to rehabilitate patients with swallowing disorders.

Throughout this book the multidisciplinary team approach to management of the dysphagic patient is stressed. The swallowing therapist and radiologist jointly perform the radiographic examination. Physicians and swallowing therapists interact in decision making regarding the time to initiate or withdraw non-oral feeding methods, as well as indications for medical vs. exercise regimens in the management of swallowing disorders. During dysphagia therapy with hospitalized patients, the nurse plays an important role in the reinforcement of management procedures with the patient. Cooperation of the physician, dietician, nurse, and swallowing therapist ensures the availability of the correct food consistencies to facilitate each patient's oral intake and the maintenance of adequate nutrition until the patient can eat by mouth adequately.

It is anticipated that this volume will be of interest to physicians managing patients with oral feeding disorders, radiologists, and allied health professionals involved in swallowing retraining, including nurses, speech pathologists, physical therapists, dieticians, and occupational therapists. It is hoped that it will stimulate research in the diagnosis and management of dysphagia, and assist interested professionals in practical diagnosis and management of a potentially frustrating patient population—those unable to maintain adequate oral intake as the result of a variety of etiologies.

I would like to thank a number of individuals who have assisted in the production of this book and in the collection of the research data incorporated in it: to Jo Ann Willoughby, the radiology technician who has assisted me with the radiographic studies since their inception in 1972; to Suzanne Donnelly, Mary MacLean, and Liz Fitzmaurice who have tirelessly typed and retyped the manuscript, and to Candace Rupick, research assistant, who has contributed to the completion of numerous details of the manuscript. Particular thanks go to Kathy Sisson, for the artwork and to my colleagues, Hilda Fisher, Patricia Jenkins, Cathy Lazarus, Fred McConnell, Mary O'Gara, and JoAnn Robbins for endless support, patience, suggestions, and time in reading, challenging, and collaborating on the contents of this manuscript.

Jeri A. Logemann

1

Introduction

Swallowing disorders occur in all age groups from newborns to the elderly, and can occur as a result of a variety of medical conditions. They may present themselves acutely, for example as a result of cerebrovascular accident (CVA) or may worsen slowly over time as in tumors of the pharynx or progressive neurologic disease. Patients with swallowing disorders may be acutely aware of their problem, and be able to describe it to the clinician in great detail, or may be entirely oblivious to any difficulty with deglutition. Patients who do report swallowing disorders and who are able to describe them, are typically highly accurate in their localization and definition of the problem (Kirchner, 1967).

This text limits itself to discussion of the swallowing problems occurring in the preparatory, oral, and pharyngeal stages of the swallow. Swallowing disorders occurring in the esophageal stage of the swallow are not discussed in detail because they are not amenable to techniques of swallowing therapy. Similarly, the text does not cover disorders related to the presence of tumors in the oral cavity or pharynx, though effects on deglutition of treatment for oral pharyngeal cancer are outlined.

Literature on disorders of deglutition falls into three categories. There are a number of studies devoted to the physiology of normal swallowing, including assessment of the oral stage of the swallow, the swallowing reflex and its triggering mechanism, and the pharyngeal and esophageal stages of deglutition (Ardran & Kemp, 1951, 1956, 1967; Bosma, 1957, 1973; Dellow, 1976; Miller, 1972).

Another large body of research has dealt with the physiology of swallowing for a variety of medical conditions. Some of these studies focus on particular aspects of deglutition, such as the oral or the pharyngeal stage of the swallow (Linde & Westover, 1962; Sloan, 1977). Others examine a small number of patients in each of a variety of disorders and make broad comparisons of swallowing physiology between these subgroups (Conley,

3

1960; Logemann & Bytell, 1979). Still, other research examines in greater detail the swallowing physiology of a specific group of patients, such as those who have undergone hemilaryngectomy or supraglottic laryngectomy or have bulbar polio, myotonic dystrophy, or oculopharyngeal dystrophy (Duranceau, Letendre, Clermont, Levisque, & Barbeau, 1978; Kaplan, 1951; Margulies, Brunt, Donner, & Silbiger, 1968).

Finally, there is a body of information in the literature which presents methodologies for diagnosis and management of patients with dysphagia (Aguilar, Olson, & Shedd, 1979; Dobie, 1978; Gaffney & Campbell, 1974; Kirchner, 1967; Linden & Siebens, 1980). Articles in this category can be divided into two groups: Those that describe procedures to improve the oral stage of the swallow, including both manipulation of food in the preparatory stage prior to swallowing and the transport of food through the oral cavity; and articles that discuss techniques to improve the triggering of the reflexive swallow and the pharyngeal stage of the swallow, in addition to the preparatory stage of oral manipulation and the oral stage. Articles in the former group generally describe procedures that can be called *feeding techniques* while those in the latter category describe methodologies for *swallowing therapy*.

Feeding vs. Swallowing

Typically, the term *feeding* is limited to the placement of food in the mouth, the manipulation of food in the oral cavity prior to the initiation of the swallow, including mastication if necessary, and the oral stage of the swallow when the bolus is propelled backward by the tongue. Therapy procedures designed to improve feeding generally include: (1) positioning of material in the mouth, (2) manipulating food in the mouth with the tongue, (3) chewing a bolus of varying consistencies, (4) recollecting the bolus into a cohesive mass prior to initiation of the swallow, and (5) organizing lingual peristalsis to propel the bolus posteriorly. Thus, feeding techniques deal with the preparatory and oral stages of the swallow that terminate when the reflexive swallow is triggered.

In contrast, procedures used in swallowing therapy include techniques for stimulation of the swallowing reflex, improvement of pharyngeal transit time and airway protection, as well as all of the techniques used to improve the preparatory and oral stage of the swallow. Thus, the term *swallowing* refers to the entire act of deglutition from placement of food in the mouth through the oral and pharyngeal stages of the swallow until the material enters the esophagus through the cricopharyngeal juncture. Throughout this book, the term swallowing rather than feeding will be used, as the physiology of deglutition will be examined in all stages and techniques for modification of disorders in each stage of the swallow will be discussed.

Multidisciplinary Approach

The approach to management of swallowing disorders discussed here represents a multidisciplinary model for the safe evaluation and treatment of patients with a swallowing problem that makes oral feeding difficult or impossible. The dysphagia team includes the patient's physician(s), nursing staff, dietician, and radiologist, in addition to the swallowing therapist. Although the bedside examination is conducted by the swallowing therapist, the radiographic examination is usually conducted by both the radiologist and the swallowing therapist (usually the speech pathologist), and resulting chart notes and recommendations are the consensus of the two professionals. Once a management program has been outlined by the swallowing therapist in conjunction with the patient's attending physician, the swallowing therapist typically involves the nursing staff for day-to-day carryover of desired procedures, and interacts closely with the dietician to insure adequate nutrition throughout the program. The philosophy reiterated throughout this book is that swallowing therapy is superimposed on continuously adequate nutrition. Nutrition is never jeopardized during the course of management of the patient's swallowing problem. Thus, from the day of the initial evaluation, the swallowing therapist must interact closely with the patient's physician, nursing staff, and dietician to outline the best program to maintain nutrition and increasingly improve the patient's swallowing function.

Patient Safety

A concern second only to maintenance of adequate nutrition in the management of a patient with difficulty in swallowing is safety of the patient during oral feedings. In general, aspiration (entry of material into the airway below the true vocal cords) should be kept to a minimum. Currently, there are no clear guidelines as to the amount of aspiration which can be tolerated by a patient before such complications as aspiration pneumonia arise. And the interaction between such parameters as pulmonary function and tolerance for aspiration are not clearly understood. Aspiration is kept to a minimum by giving the patient only a small amount of material during the bedside clinical and radiographic examinations and by determining radiographically the gross amount of aspiration the patient experiences per bolus. Any patient whose aspiration is larger than approximately 10% per bolus of a particular food consistency should be restricted from eating that consistency of food by mouth. This recommendation is based on data collected from 50 surgically treated head and neck cancer patients who aspirated food postoperatively. All of these patients were aware of the aspiration after it entered their airway below the vocal cords, and were able to expectorate most of the aspirated material. These patients spontaneously stopped eating the food consistencies on which they had aspiration greater than approximately 10% because the continuous coughing quickly became uncomfortable. Patients who could not swallow any food consistency without more than approximately 10% aspiration stopped eating all foods by mouth and required nasogastric feedings (Logemann, Sisson, & Wheeler, 1980). Many physicians consider chronic aspiration of more than small trace amounts (liquid or solid) as a hazard to normal pulmonary function. Others are more tolerant of larger amounts of aspiration for short periods of time. This variance results from each physician's individual experience and the absence of clear guidelines for management beyond those presented above.

It is equally important to insure that a patient's airway not be blocked by a bolus of material that may be entirely aspirated. Thus, throughout this text you will find frequent references to the use of small amounts of material, i.e. ⅓ teaspoon or approximately 2 cc, insufficient to ever completely block or even severely narrow a patient's airway.

The patient's safety during swallowing therapy can also be assured by completing a radiographic diagnostic examination in addition to any bedside clinical evaluation. A radiographic examination will identify any silent aspirators, i.e. those patients whose sensitivity is reduced and who aspirate food or liquid without coughing or other visible or audible sign. Research has shown that even the most experienced clinicians will fail to identify approximately 40% of the patients who aspirate during a bedside examination (Logemann, Lazarus, & Jenkins, 1982). Therefore, radiographic evaluation of any patient who is suspected of aspiration is absolutely necessary to identify the presence of aspiration, to define the etiology of the aspiration, to design appropriate therapy for the patient, and to determine the best method of nutritional intake.

Bibliography

Aguilar, N., Olson, M., & Shedd, D. Rehabilitation of deglutition problems in patients with head and neck cancer. *American Journal of Surgery*, 1979, *138*, 501–507.

Ardran, G., & Kemp, F. The mechanism of swallowing. *Proceedings of the Royal Society of Medicine*, 1951, *44*, 1038–1040.

Ardran, G., & Kemp, F. Closure and opening of the larynx during swallowing. *British Journal of Radiology*, 1956, *29*, 205–208.

Ardran, G., & Kemp, F. The mechanism of the larynx II. The epiglottis and closure of the larynx. *British Journal of Radiology*, 1967, *40*, 372–389.

Bosma, J. Deglutition: Pharyngeal stage. *Physiological Reviews*, 1957, *37*, 275–300.

Bosma, J. Physiology of the mouth, pharynx and esophagus. In M. Paparella & D. Shumrick (Eds.), *Otolaryngology volume 1: Basic sciences and related disciplines.* Philadelphia: W. B. Saunders, 1973, 356–370.

Conley, J. Swallowing dysfunctions associated with radical surgery of the head and neck. *Archives of Surgery*, 1960, *80*, 602–612.

Dellow, P. The general physiological background of chewing and swallowing. In B. Sessle & A. Hannan (Eds.), *Mastication and swallowing.* Toronto: University of Toronto Press, 1976.

Dobie, R. Rehabilitation of swallowing disorders. *American Family Physician*, 1978, *17*, 84–95.

Duranceau, C., Letendre, J., Clermont, R., Levisque, H., & Barbeau, A. Oropharyngeal dysphagia in patients with oculopharyngeal muscular dystrophy. *Canadian Journal of Surgery*, 1978, *21*, 326–329.

Gaffney, T., & Campbell, R. Feeding techniques for dysphagic patients. *American Journal of Nursing*, 1974, *74*, 2194–2195.

Kaplan, S. Paralysis of deglutition. A post poly-poliomyelitis complication treated by sections of the cricopharyngeus muscle. *Annals of Surgery*, 1951, *133*, 572–573.

Kirchner, J. Pharyngeal and esophageal dysfunction: The diagnosis. *Minnesota Medicine*, 1967, *50*, 921–924.

Linde, L., & Westover, J. Esophageal and gastric abnormalities in dysautonomia. *Pediatrics*, 1962, *29*, 303–306.

Linden, P., & Siebens, A. Videofluoroscopy: Use in evaluation and treatment of dysphagia. Miniseminar presented at the American Speech Language Hearing Association annual meeting in Detroit, November 1980.

Logemann, J., & Bytell, D. Swallowing disorders in three types of head and neck surgical patients. *Cancer,* 1979, *44,* 1075–1105.

Logemann, J., Lazarus, C., & Jenkins, P. The relationship between clinical judgment and radiographic assessment of aspiration. Paper presented at the American Speech Language Hearing Association annual meeting, Toronto, November 1982.

Logemann, J., Sisson, G., & Wheeler, R. The team approach to rehabilitation of surgically treated oral cancer patients. *Proceedings of the National Forum on Cancer Rehabilitation,* 1980, Williamsburg, VA, 222–227.

Margulies, S., Brunt, P., Donner, M., & Silbiger, M. Familial dysautonomia. A cineradiographic study of the swallowing mechanism. *Radiology,* 1968, *90,* 107–112.

Miller, A. Characteristics of the swallowing reflex induced by peripheral nerve and brain stem stimulation. *Experimental Neurology,* 1972, *34,* 210–222.

Sloan. R. Cinefluorographic study of cerebral palsy deglutition. *Journal of the Osaka Dental University,* 1977, *11,* 58–73.

2

Anatomy and Physiology of Normal Deglutition

Anatomic Structures

The anatomic areas involved in deglutition include the oral cavity, pharynx, larynx, and esophagus, shown in midsaggittal section in Figure 2-1. Structures in the oral cavity are labeled in Figures 2-1 and 2-2, and include the lips anteriorly, the teeth (24 deciduous teeth, 32 permanent teeth), hard palate, soft palate, uvula, mandible or lower jaw, floor of mouth, tongue, and faucial arches. Between the anterior and posterior faucial arches are the palatine tonsils, as seen in Figure 2-2, easily viewed during an oral examination. In patients with swallowing disorders, the pockets or side cavities created by the normal juxtaposition of structures often play a key role in the lodging or pocketing of material. For example, the sulcus is the space formed between the alveolus and cheek or lip musculature. Thus, there are sulci around the maxilla and mandible, both laterally and anteriorly, as shown in Figure 2-3.

Pharyngeal structures involved in deglutition include the three pharyngeal constrictors, superior, medial, and inferior. As pictured in Figure 2-4, fibers comprising these muscles arise from the median raphe in the midline of the posterior pharyngeal wall, and run laterally to attach to boney and soft tissue structures located anteriorly. Structures to which these fibers attach include the pterygoid plates on the sphenoid bone, the soft palate, the base of the tongue, the mandible, the hyoid bone, and the thyroid and cricoid cartilages. As the fibers of the inferior constrictor attach to the sides of the thyroid cartilage anteriorly, a space is formed between these fibers and the sides of the thyroid cartilage, as illustrated in Figure 2-5. These spaces are known as the pyriform sinuses. These end inferiorly at the cricopharyngeus muscle, which is the most inferior structure of the pharynx, and in fact, serves as the valve at the top of the

11

FIGURE 2-1
Mid-sagittal section of the head and neck.

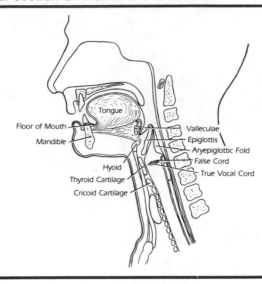

Tongue

Floor of Mouth

Mandible

Valleculae

Epiglottis

Aryepiglottic Fold

False Cord

Hyoid

True Vocal Cord

Thyroid Cartilage

Cricoid Cartilage

FIGURE 2-2
Frontal view of the oral cavity, showing anterior and posterior faucial arches.

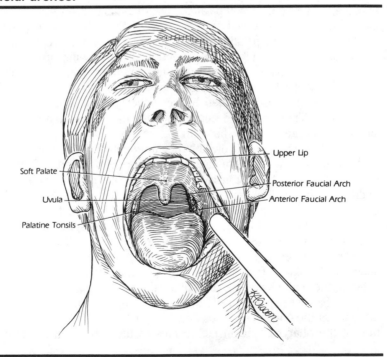

Soft Palate

Uvula

Palatine Tonsils

Upper Lip

Posterior Faucial Arch

Anterior Faucial Arch

FIGURE 2-3
Frontal view of the oral cavity with the lower lip pulled outward to reveal the anterior and lateral sulci.

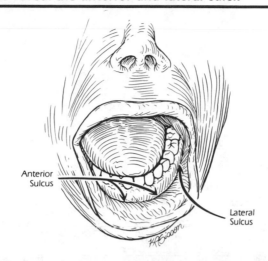

Anterior Sulcus

Lateral Sulcus

FIGURE 2-4
Lateral view of the pharyngeal constrictors (superior, medial and inferior) and their anterior attachments.

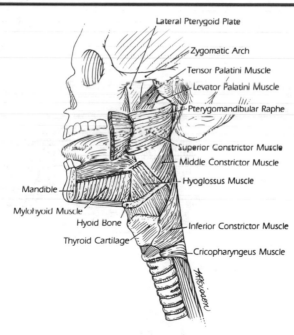

Lateral Pterygoid Plate

Zygomatic Arch

Tensor Palatini Muscle

Levator Palatini Muscle

Pterygomandibular Raphe

Superior Constrictor Muscle

Middle Constrictor Muscle

Hyoglossus Muscle

Mandible

Mylohyoid Muscle

Hyoid Bone

Thyroid Cartilage

Inferior Constrictor Muscle

Cricopharyngeus Muscle

FIGURE 2-5 (a, b)
Posterior views of the pharynx with the pharyngeal constrictors cut at midline and laid back to reveal the strictures anterior to the pharynx. The pyriform sinuses can be seen as spaces created between the sides of the larynx and the pharyngeal constrictors. Arrows on Figure (a) indicate the pathway of food and liquid down the pyriform sinuses on each side during the swallow.

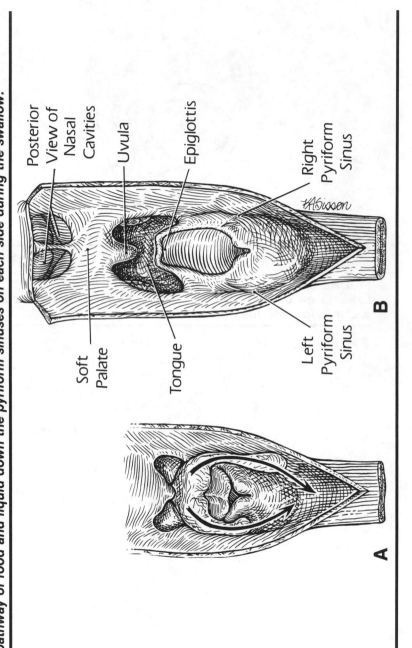

Soft Palate

Posterior View of Nasal Cavities

Uvula

Epiglottis

Right Pyriform Sinus

Left Pyriform Sinus

Tongue

tASissen

B

A

esophagus. These muscle fibers have been described by some investigators as part of the inferior constrictor. At rest, these fibers (also known as the pharyngoesophageal juncture or P-E segment) are in tonic contraction to prevent air from entering the esophagus during respiration and material from refluxing back up the esophagus and into the pharynx (Kirchner, 1958; Parrish, 1968). The fibers create a 2 to 4 cm zone of elevated pressure capable of withstanding pressures of up to 11 cm of water in the esophagus. The cricopharyngeal sphincter has greatest pressure immediately prior to the swallow and during inspiration. Increase in pressure during inhalation insures that no air is pulled into the esophagus (Parrish, 1968). At the appropriate moment during swallowing, the fibers relax to allow the bolus to pass into the esophagus.

The esophagus consists of a hollow muscular tube approximately 23 to 25 cm long with a sphincter at each end. It has two layers of muscle, the inner circular, the outer longitudinal. Each layer is made up of striated muscle in the upper third, a combination of striated and smooth muscle in the middle third, and smooth muscle in lower one third (Hansky, 1973; Ponzoli, 1968).

At the base of the tongue, the pharynx opens into the larynx, which is designed primarily as a valve to keep food from entering the airway during swallowing as shown in Figure 2-1. The topmost structure of the larynx is the epiglottis, which rests against the base of the tongue. The wedge-shaped space formed between the base of the tongue and epiglottis is the valleculae. Together, the valleculae and the pyriform sinuses are known as the pharyngeal recesses or side pockets, into which food may fall and reside before or after the swallowing reflex triggers. The lingual tonsils are located against the base of the tongue and take up a small amount of the vallecular space. The opening into the larynx (the area posterior and inferior to the epiglottis) is known as the laryngeal vestibule, which ends at the superior surface of the false vocal folds.

The intrinsic structures of the larynx are shown in Figures 2-6 and 2-7. The aryepiglottic folds, containing the aryepiglottic muscle, quadrangular membrane and cuneiform cartilages, are attached to the lateral margins of the epiglottis and run laterally, posteriorly, and inferiorly to surround the arytenoid cartilages. The two arytenoids are positioned on the rim of the cricoid cartilage posteriorly. Muscular pull on these arytenoid cartilages controls movement of the true vocal cords. The posterior cricoarytenoid muscle, attaching from the posterior surface of the cricoid lamina to the muscular process of the arytenoid, opens or abducts the true vocal folds. The lateral cricoarytenoid (attaching from the top edge of the cricoid cartilage at the side to the muscular process of the arytenoid) and the interarytenoid muscles (attaching between the two arytenoid cartilages) adduct or close the vocal cords across the top of the airway (Pressman & Kelemen, 1955).

FIGURE 2-6
Superior view of the intrinsic laryngeal structures.

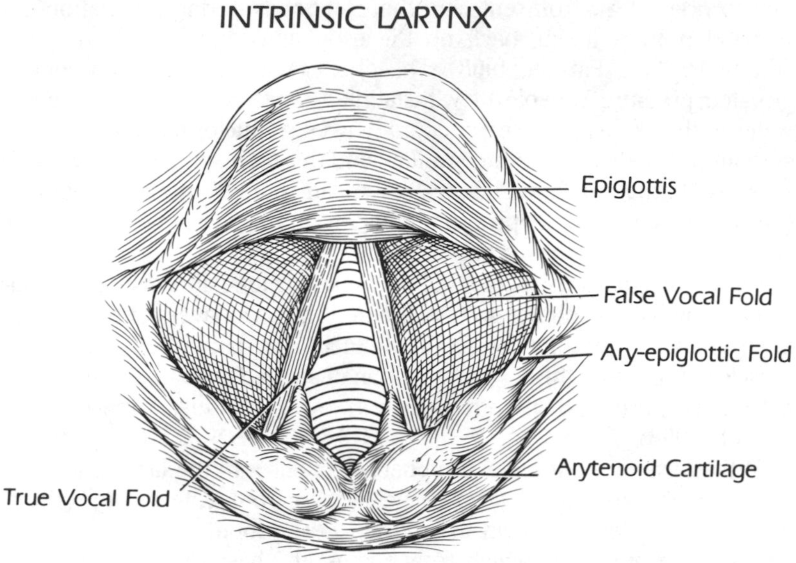

INTRINSIC LARYNX

As shown in Figure 2-7, the aryepiglottic folds end inferiorly in the false vocal folds, two shelves of muscle and connective tissue running anteriorly to posteriorly immediately above the level of the true vocal cords. The true vocal folds, composed of vocalis and thyroarytenoid muscles, are attached to the vocal process of the arytenoids posteriorly, to the inside surface of the thyroid lamina laterally, and to the thyroid notch anteriorly. These, then, form two more shelves of soft tissue that when adducted or closed, project into the airway and effectively close the top of the trachea. The false vocal cords parallel the true vocal cords superiorly. Like the true cords, the false vocal cords form shelves of soft tissue projecting from the sides of the larynx, anteriorly to posteriorly. The space that is formed between the false and true vocal cords on each side is known as the laryngeal ventricle. Together the epiglottis and aryepiglottic folds, false vocal folds, and true vocal folds form three levels of sphincter at the top of the trachea, capable of completely closing it off from the pharynx and preventing penetration of food or liquid during swallowing (Lederman, 1977; Pressman & Kelemen, 1955).

The larynx and trachea are suspended in the neck between the hyoid bone superiorly and the sternum inferiorly, as shown in Figure 2-8. A number of muscles, categorized as the laryngeal strap muscles, contribute

FIGURE 2-7 (a, b)
Frontal (a) and lateral (b) views of intrinsic structures of the larynx.

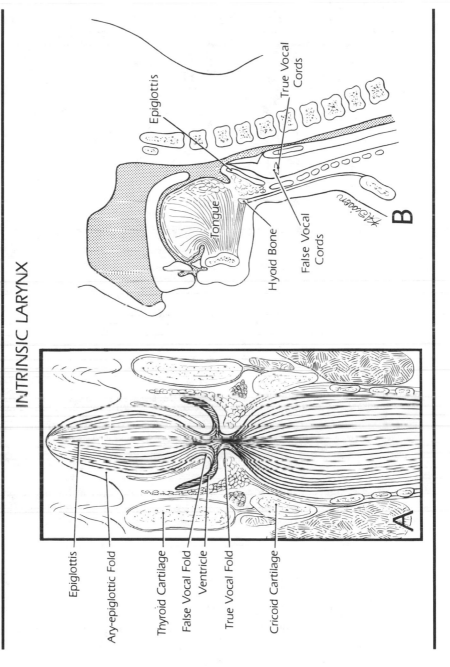

INTRINSIC LARYNX

FIGURE 2-8
Frontal-lateral view of the strap muscles suspending the larynx in the neck between the hyoid bone and the sternum.

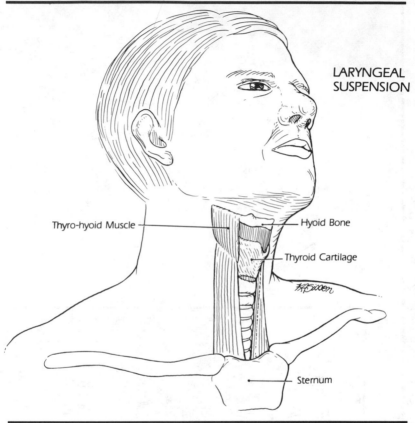

LARYNGEAL
SUSPENSION

Thyro-hyoid Muscle

Hyoid Bone

Thyroid Cartilage

Sternum

to this suspension and, together with the elasticity in the trachea itself, permit the larynx to be elevated and lowered for various activities. The hyoid bone also serves as the base for the tongue, which rests on it.

The Physiology

The act of deglutition can be divided into four phases: (1) the oral preparatory phase, when food is manipulated in the mouth and masticated if necessary; (2) the oral or voluntary phase of the swallow, when the tongue propels food posteriorly until the swallowing reflex is triggered; (3) the pharyngeal phase, when the reflexive swallow carries the bolus through the pharynx; and (4) the esophageal phase, when esophageal peristalsis carries the bolus through the cervical and thoracic esophagus into the stomach.

The frequency of deglutition varies with activity (Lear, Flanagan, & Moorrees, 1965; Logan, Kavanagh, & Wornall, 1967). Swallowing frequency is greatest during eating and least during sleep with other activities taking an intermediate place. Mean deglutition frequency is approximately 580 swallows per day. Records during sleep have shown periods of 20 minutes or more when no swallow occurs.

Swallowing and respiration are reciprocal functions, i.e. respiration halts during deglutition. Storey (1976) describes swallowing as an airway protective reflex because of this reciprocity.

Oral Preparatory Phase

Movement patterns in the oral preparatory phase of the swallow vary, depending on the consistency of material swallowed and the amount of oral manipulation the individual uses in savoring the particular food. From the time the material is placed in the mouth, labial seal is maintained to ensure that no food or liquid falls from the mouth. During liquid swallows, oral manipulation of the bolus will vary greatly from individual to individual. When placed into the mouth, a liquid bolus has a certain degree of cohesiveness that may be maintained as the bolus is held between the tongue and the anterior hard palate in preparation for the swallow. In this case, the tongue may cup around the liquid bolus and seal it against the hard palate. Some individuals may desire to move the liquid around in the mouth prior to swallowing it, and may in the process spread the bolus evenly or unevenly throughout the oral cavity. However, prior to initiating the swallow, the material is generally pulled together into a cohesive bolus by the tongue, and held between the tongue and anterior palate. Holding the bolus more anteriorly between the tongue and the anterior teeth is an abnormal preswallow position in adults, and often indicates that a tongue thrust oral swallowing pattern will be used. The tongue thrust pattern, in which the tongue moves anteriorly with the bolus before moving posteriorly, is often seen in adults with frontal lobe damage.

Oral manipulation of paste consistency materials again depends somewhat upon the preference of the individual. As with liquids, the material is introduced into the oral cavity as a cohesive bolus. In preparation for the swallow it may be maintained as such, and held on the tongue or between the tongue and hard palate, with the sides of the tongue sealed around the maxillary alveolus. Or, the individual may choose to manipulate the bolus in the mouth, lateralize it, masticate it somewhat by moving the mandible and tongue in a lateral rotary motion before bringing the material into a cohesive bolus and initiating the swallow. The cohesiveness of the paste bolus during and after entry into the oral cavity sometimes makes patients with reduced tongue control prefer this consistency. However, if the consistency of the paste is too thick, it may be more difficult for the individual with reduced tongue control to propel the material posteriorly and to keep it from adhering to the hard palate.

The oral preparatory phase of deglutition for materials requiring mastication involves a rotary lateral movement of the mandible and tongue. When the upper and lower teeth have met and crushed the material, it falls medially toward the tongue, which moves the material back onto the teeth as the mandible opens. The cycle is repeated numerous times before initiating the swallow. In addition to this cyclic movement during mastication, the tongue mixes food with saliva (Lowe, 1981). It has been postulated that the rhythmical movements of mastication are controlled by a central pattern generator. In addition, peripheral feedback is important in positioning the bolus on the teeth and preventing injury to the tongue during chewing (Lowe, 1981). Tension in the buccal musculature closes off the lateral sulcus and prevents food particles from falling into the sulcus between the mandible and the cheek (Bosma, 1973). Rotary tongue and jaw motion is continued until the swallow is about to be initiated, when material that has been masticated is again pulled together into a semicohesive bolus before the swallow is initiated. In some normal individuals, masticated materials spread more broadly throughout the oral cavity, and some portion of the bolus collects on the posterior tongue, beginning entry into the pharynx before initiation of the voluntary swallow.

During the oral preparatory phase, the velum is normally pulled actively anteriorly and rests against the back of the tongue, which is elevated somewhat, serving to keep material in the oral cavity (Fletcher, 1974; Negus, 1949; Robbins, Logemann, & Kirshner, 1982; Storey, 1976; Shedd, Scatliff, & Kirchner, 1960; Wildman, 1976). This active lowering and anterior bulging of the soft palate results from contraction of the palatoglossus muscle. The larynx and pharynx are at rest during the preparatory phase of swallowing. The airway is open and nasal breathing may continue until the voluntary swallow is initiated. Clearly, if an individual loses control of a part of the bolus during this oral preparatory phase and it trickles into the pharynx, the material may continue to drop down and enter the open airway. The reflexive swallow rarely triggers in response to this material, possibly because the voluntary swallow has not been initiated.

In summary, immediately before initiation of the oral or voluntary stage of the swallow, the major portion of the bolus is pulled together into a cohesive mass and held between the anterior tongue and the palate, with the tongue cupping around the bolus and sealing it against the hard palate, laterally and anteriorly.

The sequence of the movements of the upper aerodigestive tract during deglutition are illustrated in Figure 2-9, a-e.

Oral Phase

The oral stage of the swallow is initiated when the tongue begins posterior movement of the bolus. Tongue movement during this oral phase has often been described as *stripping action,* with the tongue sequentially squeezing the bolus posteriorly against the hard palate (Ardran & Kemp, 1951; Lowe, 1981, Negus, 1949). Another way to describe this tongue movement would be as an anterior to posterior rolling action, with tongue elevation progressing sequentially more posteriorly to push the bolus backward. During this time a central groove is formed, acting as a ramp, or chute, for food to pass through as it moves posteriorly (Ramsey, Watson, Gramiak, & Weinberg, 1955; Shedd et al., 1960). Several authors have described the contribution of negative pressure created by slight inward movement and increased tension of the buccal musculature in propelling the bolus posteriorly (Shedd, Kirchner & Scatliff, 1961). At the point where the bolus passes the anterior faucial arches, the oral stage of the swallow is terminated and the swallowing reflex is triggered. The oral stage of the swallow typically takes less than one second to complete and is generally considered to be the voluntary stage of the swallow. Some investigators feel that initiation of the voluntary stage of the swallow contributes to triggering the reflexive swallow, and without attempts to voluntarily initiate the swallow, reflexive triggering may be delayed or reduced.

In summary, the oral stage of the swallow involves intact labial musculature to insure an adequate seal to prevent material from leaking from

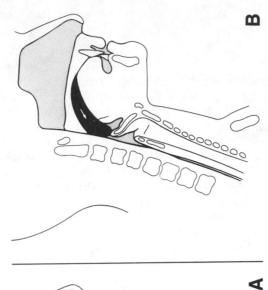

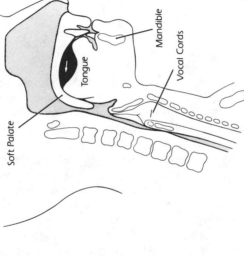

FIGURE 2-9 (a-e)
Lateral view of bolus propulsion during the swallow, beginning with the voluntary initiation of the swallow by the tongue (a); the triggering of the swallowing reflex (b); the bolus passage through the pharynx (c); the entry of the bolus through the cricopharyngeal sphincter into the cervical esophagus (d); and the completion of the pharyngeal stage of the swallow when the entire bolus is in the cervical esophagus (e).

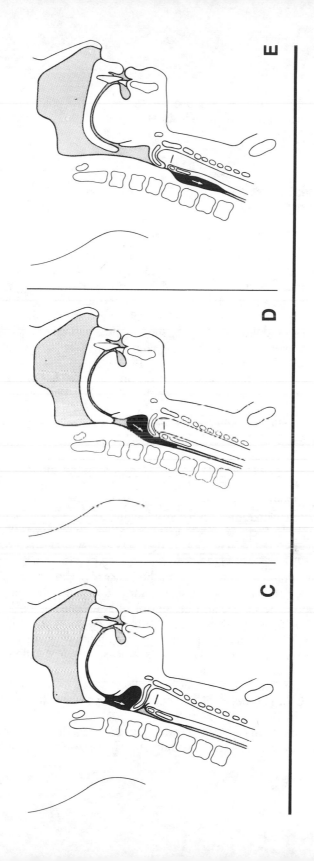

C

D

E

the oral cavity, intact lingual movement to propel the bolus posteriorly, and intact buccal musculature to insure that material does not fall into the lateral sulci.

Pharyngeal Phase—
Swallowing Reflex

The pharyngeal stage of the swallow begins with the triggering of the swallowing reflex. In the normal individual, triggering of the swallowing reflex occurs at the anterior faucial arch and timing of the reflex is such that posterior movement of the bolus is not interrupted (Jean & Car, 1979; Lederman, 1977). There is no pause in bolus movement while the reflex triggers. Pommerenke's study, published in 1928 and others have established the base of the anterior faucial pillars as the most sensitive place for elicitation of this reflex. Hollshwandner, Brenman, and Friedman in 1975 and Storey in 1976 postulated receptors in the tongue, epiglottis, and larynx, respectively, as additional centers for elicitation of the reflex. Observations of neurologically impaired patients by this author corroborate these variations. Some patients do not trigger a reflex until the bolus has contacted the aryepiglottic folds, while others trigger the reflex only when material has fallen into the pyriform sinuses.

Dobie (1978), Donner and Silbiger (1966), Cumming and Reilly (1972), and others have suggested that the sensory portion of the swallowing reflex is carried by cranial nerves IX, X, and XI. The impulses travel to the medullary reticular formation, or swallowing center, located within the brainstem (Doty, Richmond, & Storey 1967; Miller, 1972; Sumi, 1972). This center acts as a neuronal pool to organize the synergy necessary for normal swallowing. The motor portion is carried by IX and X. The VIIth nerve may additionally contribute to the sensory portion. Nerves V, VII, and XII have been named as possible contributors to the afferent portion.

The role of the cerebellum in control of swallowing is unclear. The work of Brooks, Kozlovskaya, Atkin, Horvath, & Uno (1973), Kent and Netsell (1975), and Larson and Sutton (1978) indicates cerebellar input into the velocity of movement and, thus, at least into mastication and the preparatory phase of the swallow.

Cortical input into the control of swallowing is not well understood, although abnormal swallowing is observed in patients after damage to cortical areas.

There is much which is not known about the triggering of the swallowing reflex. However, it is clear that humans cannot swallow unless there is something in their mouth, either food, liquid, or saliva. If one attempts to swallow four times in rapid succession, it is difficult to continue past the second or third swallow because these dry swallows have depleted saliva in the mouth.

There is, no doubt, a relationship between voluntary attempts to swallow and triggering of the swallowing reflex. The exact nature of that relationship, however, is not understood. It is clear that simply placing food or liquid in the mouth will not trigger the reflex unless there is the voluntary initiation of swallowing. Direct stimulation to the areas where the swallowing reflex is triggered using a light touch or stronger stimulation will usually not stimulate the swallow unless saliva or other material is present and the patient is also attempting voluntarily to initiate the swallow. Roueche (1980) probably states it best, ". . . both voluntary and reflex components are involved in the normal swallow. Neither mechanism alone is capable of producing swallowing with the regularity and immediacy which is necessary during the normal process of oral feeding."

Triggering of the swallowing reflex causes a number of physiological activities to occur simultaneously. These are critical to successful swallowing and include: (1) elevation and retraction of the velum and complete closure of the velopharyngeal port to prevent material from entering the nasal cavity; (2) initiation of pharyngeal peristalsis to pick up the bolus as it passes the anterior faucial arch and carry it by sequential peristaltic (squeezing) action of the pharyngeal constrictors into and through the pharynx to the cricopharyngeal sphincter at the top of the esophagus; (3) elevation and closure of the larynx at all three sphincters (epiglottis/aryepiglottic folds, false vocal folds, and true vocal folds) to prevent material from entering the airway; and (4) relaxation of the cricopharyngeal sphincter to allow material to pass from the pharynx into the esophagus.

Ardran and Kemp (1952, 1956) describe the closure of the larynx as extending from the level of the vocal cords to the laryngeal vestibule. These researchers' cineradiographic studies indicate that closure is effected from below upwards, with the contents of the laryngeal vestibule being expressed into the pharynx. During closure, there is a downward, forward, and inward rocking movement of the arytenoid cartilages which narrows the laryngeal opening (Ardran & Kemp, 1967). At the same time the larynx is elevated and pulled forward, its opening is arched backwards (Ardran & Kemp, 1956; Negus, 1949).

Without the triggering of the swallowing reflex, none of the four physiologic activities listed occur. If the tongue propels the bolus posteriorly and no reflex is triggered, the bolus is likely to be propelled by the tongue into the pharynx, where it may come to rest in the valleculae. If the material is liquid, it may splash into the pharynx and into the open airway. No pharyngeal activity will occur until the swallowing reflex triggers, so the bolus may rest in the valleculae until the reflex is triggered. Or, depending on consistency, the food may drain from the valleculae down the aryepiglottic folds and into the pyriform sinus, or may fall into the airway where it may or may not be expectorated, depending upon the patient's sensitivity in the trachea and larynx. It is important to remember that velar, pharyngeal, and laryngeal activity occur only as a result of the reflex. Patients can be taught to voluntarily protect their airway, as described in Chapter 5; but there is no way to voluntarily initiate or modify pharyngeal peristalsis or velopharyngeal closure during swallowing (Hollis & Castell, 1975). There is some question as to whether patients can learn to relax the cricopharyngeus muscle voluntarily, as seen in sword swallowers (Devgan, Bross, McCloy, & Smith, 1978) and some alaryngeal speakers.

Pharyngeal transit time, the time taken for the bolus to move from the point at which the reflex is triggered at the anterior faucial arch through the cricopharyngeal juncture into the esophagus, is normally one second or less. Normally, during this transit, the bolus does not hesitate anywhere in the pharynx, but moves smoothly and quickly over the base of the tongue through the pharynx and into the cervical esophagus. As the bolus moves through the pharynx, it usually divides, with approximately half flowing down each side of the pharynx through the pyriform sinuses. The two portions of the bolus join again at about the level of the opening of the esophagus (Ardran & Kemp, 1951). When the pharyngeal phase of the swallow is over, there is normally very little food left in the pharynx.

Esophageal Phase

Esophageal transit times can be measured from the point where the bolus enters the esophagus at the cricopharyngeal juncture until it passes into the stomach at the gastro-esophageal juncture. Normal esophageal transit time varies from 8 to 20 seconds. The peristaltic wave which begins in the pharynx when the swallowing reflex triggers, continues in sequential fashion through the esophagus.

Motility disorders in the esophagus can be defined during a videofluoroscopic study, as described in Chapter 4. However, because the esophageal phase of the swallow is not amenable to any kind of therapeutic exercise regimen, the videofluoroscopic study of deglutition generally does not involve examination of the esophagus. Patients with esophageal disorders should receive a standard barium swallow or upper GI series.

Changes with Age

Swallowing in Infancy

According to Dellow (1976), swallowing begins in the fetus, with sucking movements, drinking of amniotic fluid, and occasional presentation with the thumb in the mouth. Infant swallowing patterns differ from that of adults' in several respects. Because the size of the oral cavity is much smaller, the tongue fills the mouth and rests more anteriorly than in adults. There is also approximation of the soft palate, tongue and epiglottis, so that quiet respiration is usually nasal (Bosma, 1973; Fletcher, 1974). Initially, sucking is accomplished by downward movement of the mandible with the mouth closed, creating a drop in intra-oral pressure. This is followed by an elevation of the tongue and jaw against the maxilla and a stiffened upper lip, which pumps liquid from the nipple. As the stream of liquid reaches the posterior oral cavity, the posterior pharyngeal wall, soft palate, and base of tongue come together to propel the bolus through the pharynx. Anterior movement of the posterior pharyngeal wall is much greater in infants than adults. The larynx is much higher in infancy, and the pharynx much shorter, so that the larynx elevates to a much lesser degree in infants than adults. During postnatal development, the pharynx lengthens and enlarges, the larynx lowers, and the mandible and the hyoid descend (Bosma, 1973).

According to Bosma (1973), bite is achieved at approximately 7 months, and chewing begins at approximately 10 to 12 months.

Swallowing with Aging

There have been few studies of the changes in swallowing patterns throughout adulthood. Feldman, Kapur, Alman, and Chauncy (1980) studied masticatory function in older adults. High masticatory performance was maintained regardless of age in individuals with complete, or almost complete, dentition. These authors did find an increase in the number of chewing strokes used to prepare food for swallowing related to age and dentition status. Those studies which have examined swallowing disorders in aging adults (Mandelstam & Lieber, 1964; Blonsky, Logemann,

Boshes, & Fisher (1975) have shown that few changes in the physiology of deglutition occur until individuals reach their 80s. At that time, some reduction in the strength of pharyngeal peristalsis is seen, resulting in some residual material in the pharynx after the swallow, but no changes in the oral phase of the swallow have been noted. In these aged adults, esophageal peristalsis is also reduced with an increase in esophageal transit time.

Study Techniques

A number of techniques have been used to define and study the various stages in the swallowing act.

Radiographic Procedures

Radiographic procedures have been used to study swallowing since the early 1900s. In the 1930s, the development of fluoroscopy permitted examination of the movement patterns of the oral cavity, pharynx, and esophagus during swallowing. The fluoroscopic image, first recorded on movie film and called *cinefluoroscopy,* allowed examination of movement patterns of the bolus and of particular structures in slow motion and frame-by-frame. The movie film could be exposed at various speeds up to 60 frames per second. (Ardran & Kemp, 1951, 1952, 1956; Sloan, Ricketts, Brummett, Bench & Westover, 1965; Sokol, Heitmann, Wolf, & Cohen, 1966; Wictorin, Hedegard, & Lundberg, 1971).

More recently, fluoroscopic studies have been recorded on videotape (videofluoroscopy), which also permits frame-by-frame analysis employing a video recorder-player with frame-by-frame analysis capability (Yotsuya, Nonaka, & Yoshinobu, 1981; Yotsuya, Saito, & Yoshinobu, 1981). By recording numbers on each frame of the videotape using a video counter timer, the swallowing studies can be repeatedly examined in slow motion or frame-by-frame, and the specific frame numbers of greatest interest can be easily located and examined. Because swallowing occurs very rapidly, with normal oral and pharyngeal transit times each taking a maximum of 1 second, slow motion analysis is most helpful in defining movement disorders. Almost any videotape recorder can be attached to the fluoroscopic equipment so that the fluoroscopic image can be easily recorded on videotape. Thus, no special equipment is generally necessary. Videofluoroscopic studies provide information on transit times, motility problems, and amount and etiology of aspiration.

Manometry

Manometric studies of swallowing have revealed a great deal of information on the pattern of the peristaltic pressure waves during deglutition. During manometry, one or more pressure-sensitive tubes of small diameter are swallowed by the patient (Fyke & Code, 1955; Kelley, 1970; Sokol et al., 1966; Vantrappen & Hellemans, 1967). In place, the tubes are sensitive to the changing pressures in the pharynx and esophagus as the patient swallows. Frequently, three tubes are positioned so that one gauge measures pressures in the upper esophageal sphincter, or the cricopharyngeus muscle, the second gauge measuring pressure within the esophagus, and the third tube measuring pressures in the lower esophageal sphincter, or the gastroesophageal juncture. The patient is asked to swallow repeatedly with the tubes in place, and the measured pressure changes are recorded on a write-out device. Using manometry, Fyke and Code (1955) identified the cricopharyngeus as a 3 cm band of high pressure at the level of the cricoid cartilage that relaxed during swallowing. At the same time the pressure dropped at the cricopharyngeus, these authors noted an increase in pressure in the upper part of the pharynx, and attributed both the pressure drop and the pressure increase to the triggering of the swallowing reflex. Dodds, Hogan, Reid, Stewart, and Arndorfer, 1973, found stronger peristalsis in the esophagus with wet swallows than dry swallows, and advocated the consistent use of wet swallows in manometric studies. Hollis and Castell (1975) also identified slower peristaltic wave speed, greater duration of the contraction wave, and later time of appearance of the peristaltic waves in the distal esophagus in a wet swallow versus a dry swallow. Patients can be asked to perform other functions with the tubes in place, such as production of esophageal voice. Also, pressure patterns in particular areas of the pharynx and esophagus can be recorded. In some cases, one gauge can be positioned in the pharynx to record pharyngeal peristalsis patterns in swallowing or other activities.

In general, esophageal manometry is used to identify disruptions in the peristaltic wave through the pharynx and esophagus and to diagnose disorders in the upper or lower esophageal sphincters (Hansky, 1973).

Manometry is frequently used in conjunction with fluoroscopy to identify esophageal disorders. Assessment of amount and etiology of aspiration is unique to fluoroscopy, and no correlation with manometric measurements is possible (Hurwitz, Nelson, & Haddad, 1975).

Electromyography

Electromyography has been frequently used to study the activity of oral musculature during deglutition, but only minimally to assess other muscle activity in humans during swallowing (Hrycyshyn & Basmajian, 1972; Ingervall, 1978). This is principally because the positioning of electrodes in the pharyngeal muscles involved in swallowing, especially the pharyngeal constrictors, is difficult. Electrodes are frequently dislodged during the muscle contraction for swallowing. Shipp, Deatsch, and Robertson (1970) studied the cricopharyngeus muscle during swallowing in humans by placing electrodes during total laryngectomy surgery.

Doty and Bosma (1956) studied reflexive deglutition in dogs, cats, and monkeys by placing two electrodes in each muscle to be analyzed. Overall, 22 muscles were examined. The swallowing reflex was activated by stimulating the pharynx with a cotton swab or rapidly injected water, or by stimulating the superior laryngeal nerve. These investigators found no difference in temporal pattern, duration, or amplitude of contraction of participating muscles in swallows elicited by these varying methods. One group of muscles (superior constrictor, palato pharyngeus, palatoglossus, posterior intrinsic muscles of the tongue, styloglossus, stylohyoid, geniohyoid, and mylohyoid) fire concurrently to initiate the swallow.

The activity of four muscles in the oral stage of the swallow was examined in humans by Hrycyshyn and Basmajian (1972). They found no universal firing pattern within the four muscles, the geniohyoid, anterior belly of digastric, mylohyoid, and genioglossus. The type of bolus appeared to affect the duration of muscle activity.

Acoustic Analyses

Several authors have examined various parameters of deglutition using acoustic procedures (Logan et al., 1967; Mackowiak, Brenman, & Friedman, 1967). Hollshwandner et al. (1975) studied some temporal measures of swallowing such as the time elapsing from the final chew of the swallowing cycle to the first sound of deglutition by attaching a contact microphone to the skin surface paralaryngeally. Using this same technique, Lear, Flanagan, and Moorrees (1965) assessed the frequency of adult deglutition over 24-hour periods. Unfortunately, acoustic techniques are limited by the few parameters of swallowing that can be studied, as many aspects of deglutition are silent.

Summary

Normal swallowing is a rapid act involving voluntary and involuntary aspects requiring complex neuromotor control. Although the exact nature of neural control is not entirely understood, the physiology of normal deglutition is clearly defined and forms a basis for comparison of the abnormalities in swallowing described in the following chapter. Of the procedures available to study deglutition, videofluoroscopy provides the greatest information on the details of physiology.

Bibliography

Ardran, G. M., & Kemp, F.   The mechanism of swallowing. *Proceedings of the Royal Society of Medicine*, 1951, *44*, 1038–1040.

Ardran, G. M., & Kemp, F.   The protection of the laryngeal airway during swallowing. *British Journal of Radiology*, 1952, *25*, 406–416.

Ardran, G., & Kemp, F.   Closure and opening of the larynx during swallowing. *British Journal of Radiology*, 1956, *29*, 205–208.

Ardran, G., & Kemp, F.   The mechanism of the larynx II. The epiglottis and closure of the larynx. *British Journal of Radiology*, 1967, *40*, 372–389.

Bieger, D., & Hockman, C.   Suprabulbar modulation of reflex swallowing. *Experimental Neurology*, 1976, *52*, 311–324.

Blonsky, E., Logemann, J., Boshes, B., & Fisher, H.   Comparison of speech and swallowing function in patients with tremor disorders and in normal geriatric patients: A cinefluorographic study. *Journal of Gerontology*, 1975, *30*, 299–303.

Bosma, J.   Deglutition: pharyngeal stage. *Physiological Reviews*, 1957, *37*, 275–300.

Bosma, J. Physiology of the mouth, pharynx and esophagus. In M. Paparella & D. Shumrick (Eds.), *Otolaryngology volume 1: Basic sciences and related disciplines.* Philadelphia: W. B. Saunders, 1973, 356–370.

Brooks, V., Kozlovskaya, I., Atkin, A., Horvath, F., & Uno, M. Effects of cooling dentate nucleus on tracking task-performance in monkeys. *Journal of Neurophysiology,* 1973, *36,* 974–995.

Burke, P. Swallowing and the organization of sucking in the human newborn. *Child Development,* 1977, *48,* 523–531.

Campbell, S. Neural control of oral somatic motor function. *Physical Therapy,* 1981, *61,* 16–22.

Cleall, J., Deglutition: A study of form and function. *American Journal of Orthodontia,* 1965, *51,* 566–594.

Cohen, M., & Levinsky, W. Topical anesthesia and swallowing. *Journal of the American Medical Association,* 1976, *236,* 562.

Cumming, W., & Reilly, B. Fatigue aspiration. *Pediatric Radiology,* 1972, *105,* 387–390.

Dellow, P. The general physiological background of chewing and swallowing. In B. Sessle & A. Hannan (Eds.), *Mastication and swallowing.* Toronto: University of Toronto Press, 1976.

Devgan, B., Bross, G., McCloy, R., & Smith, C. Anatomic and physiologic aspects of sword swallowing. *Ear, Nose and Throat,* 1978, *57,* 445–450.

Dobie, R. Rehabilitation of swallowing disorders. *American Family Physician,* 1978, *17,* 84–95.

Dodds, W., Hogan, W., Reid, D., Stewart, E., & Arndorfer, R. A comparison between primary esophageal peristalsis following wet and dry swallows. *Journal of Applied Physiology,* 1973, *35,* (6), 851–857.

Donner, M., & Silbiger, M. Cinefluorographic analysis of pharyngeal swallowing in neuromuscular disorders. *The American Journal of Medical Sciences,* 1966, *251,* 600–616.

Doty, R., & Bosma, J. An electromyographic analysis of reflex deglutition. *Journal of Neurophysiology,* 1956, *19,* 44–60.

Doty, R., Richmond, W., & Storey, A. Effect of medullary lesions on coordination of deglutition. *Experimental Neurology,* 1967, *17,* 91–106.

Feldman, R., Kapur, K., Alman, J., & Chauncey, H. H. Aging and mastication: Changes in performance and in the swallowing threshold with natural dentition. *American Geriatrics Society,* 1980, *28,* 97–103.

Fisher, M., Hendrix, T., Hurst, J., & Murrills, A. Relation between volume swallowed and velocity of the bolus ejected from the pharynx into the esophagus. *Gastroenterology,* 1978, *74,* 1238–1240.

Fletcher, S. *Tongue thrust in swallowing and speaking.* Chapter 1, The swallow pattern. Austin, TX: Learning Concepts. 1974.

Flowers, C., & Morris, H.   Oral-pharyngeal movements during swallowing and speech. *Cleft Palate Journal*, 1973, *10*, 181–191.

Frederick, J. C.   Deglutition: A study of form and function. *American Journal of Orthodontics*, 1965, *51*, 566–594.

Fyke, F., & Code, C.   Resting and deglutition pressures in the pharyngoesophageal region. *Gastroenterology*, 1955, *29*, 24–34.

Gibbs, C., Mahan, P., Lundeer, H., Brehnan, K., Walsh, E., & Holbrook, W.   Occlusal forces during chewing and swallowing as measured by sound transmission. *Journal Prosthetic Dentistry*, 1981, *46*, 443–449.

Goldberg, L.   Mononeurone mechanisms: Reflex controls. In B. Sessle and A. Hannan (Eds.), *Mastication and Swallowing*. Toronto: University of Toronto Press, 1976, 47–59.

Guelrud, M.   Swallows, wet versus dry. *Gastroenterology*, 1974, *67*, 1080–1082.

Hansky, J.   The use of oesophageal motility studies in the diagnosis of dysphagia. *Australian New Zealand Journal of Surgery*, 1973, *42*, 360–361.

Hightower, N.   New concepts of the physiology of deglutition and dysphagia. *American Journal of Surgery*, 1957, *93*, 154–161.

Hollis, J., & Castell, D.   Effect of dry and wet swallows of different volumes on esophageal peristalsis. *Journal of Applied Physiology*, 1975, *38*, 1161–1164.

Hollshwandner, G., Brenman, H., & Friedman, M.   Role of afferent sensors in the initiation of swallowing in man. *Journal of Dental Research*, 1975, *54*, 83–88.

Hoopes, J., Delton, A., Fabrikant, J., Edgerton, M. T., & Soliman, H. A.   Cineradiographic definition of the functional anatomy and pathyphysiology of the velopharynx. *Cleft Palate Journal*, 1970, *7*, 443–454.

Hrycyshyn, A., & Basmajian, J.   Electromyography of the oral stage of swallowing in man *American Journal of Anatomy*, 1972, *133*, 333–340.

Hurwitz, A., Nelson, J., & Haddad, J.   Oropharyngeal dysphagia manometric and cine esophagraphic findings. *Digestive Diseases*, 1975, *20*, 313–323.

Ingervall, B.   Activity of temporal and lip muscles during swallowing and chewing. *Journal of Oral Rehabilitation*, 1978, *5*, 329–337.

Jean, A., & Car, A.   Inputs to the swallowing medullary neurons from the peripheral afferent fibers and the swallowing cortical area. *Brain Research*, 1979, *178*, 567–572.

Jean, A., Car, A., & Roman, C.   Comparison of activity in pontine versus medullary neurones during swallowing. *Experimental Brain Research*, 1975, *22*, 211–220.

Kelley, M.   Evaluation of the patient with dysphagia. *Modern Treatment*, 1970, *27*, 1087–1097.

Kent, R., & Moll, K.   Cinefluorographic analysis of selected lingual consonants. *Journal of Speech and Hearing Research,* 1972, *15,* 453–473.

Kent, R., & Netsell, R.   A case study of an ataxic dysarthric: Cineradiographic and spectrographic observations. *Journal of Speech and Hearing Research,* 1975, *40,* 115–134.

Kirchner, J.   The motor activity of the cricopharyngeus muscle. *Laryngoscope,* 1958, *68,* 1119–1159.

Larson, C., & Sutton, D.   Effects of cerebellar lesions on monkey jaw-force control: Implications for understanding ataxic dysarthria. *Journal of Speech and Hearing Research,* 1978, *21,* 295–308.

Lear, C., Flanagan, J., & Moorrees, C.   The frequency of deglutition in man. *Archives of Oral Biology,* 1965, *10,* 83–99.

Lederman, M.   The oncology of breathing and swallowing. *Clinical Radiology,* 1977, *28,* 1–14.

Lichter, I., & Muir, R.   The pattern of swallowing during sleeping. *Electroencephalography and Clinical Neurophysiology,* 1975, *38,* 427–432.

Logan, W., Kavanagh, J., & Wornall, A.   Sonic correlates of human deglutition. *Journal of Applied Physiology,* 1967, *23,* 279–284.

Lowe, A.   The neural regulation of tongue movement. *Progress in Neurobiology,* 1981, *15,* 295–344.

Mackowiak, R., Brenman, H., & Friedman, M.   Acoustic profile of deglutition. *Proceedings of the Society for Experimental Biology,* 1967, *125,* 1149–1152.

Magoun, H.   Neurophysiology (vol. 11). In J. Field & V. Hall (Eds.), *Handbook of physiology.* Washington, DC: American Physiological Society, 1960.

Mandelstam, P., & Lieber, A.   Cineradiographic evaluation of the esophagus in normal adults. *Gastroenterology,* 1970, *58,* 32–38.

Mansson, I., & Sandberg, N.   Effects of surface anesthesia on deglutition in man. *Laryngoscope,* 1974, *84,* 427–436.

Mansson, I., & Sandberg, N.   Oropharyngeal sensitivity and elicitation of swallowing in man. *Acta Otolaryngologica,* 1975, *79,* 140–145. (a)

Mansson, I., & Sandberg, N.   Salivary stimulus and swallowing reflex in man. *Acta Otolaryngologica,* 1975, *79,* 445–450. (b)

Martensson, A.   Reflex responses and recurrent discharges evoked by stimulation of laryngeal nerves. *Acta Physiologia Scandinavia,* 1963, *57,* 248–269.

Miller, A.   Characteristics of the swallowing reflex induced by perypheral nerve and brain stem stimulation. *Experimental Neurology,* 1972, *34,* 210–222.

Miller, A., & Bowman, J.   Divergent synaptic influences affecting discharge patterning of genioglossus motor units. *Brain Research,* 1974, *78,* 179–191.

Miller, A., & Loizzi, R.   Anatomical and functional differentiation of superior laryngeal nerve fibers affecting swallowing and respiration. *Experimental Neurology,* 1974, *42,* 369–387.

Negus, V.   The second stage of swallowing. *Acta Otolaryngologica* (Supplement), 1949, 75–81, 78–82.

Nelsen, R.   Influence of chew or swallow. *Journal of the American Medical Association,* 1979, *241,* 238.

Nielsen, I., & Brenner, C.   Lower oesophageal sphincter resting pressures in achalasia and the response of the sphincter to swallowing and drugs. *South African Medical Journal,* 1976, *50,* 1822–1825.

Ogg, H.   Oral-pharyngeal development and evaluation. *Physical Therapy,* 1975, *55,* 235–241.

Parrish, R.   Cricopharyngeus dysfunction and acute dysphagia. *Canadian Medical Association Journal,* 1968, *99,* 1167–1171.

Pommerenke, W.   A study of the sensory areas eliciting the swallowing reflex. *American Journal of Physiology,* 1928, *84,* 36–41.

Ponzoli, V.   Zenker's diverticulum. *Southern Medical Journal,* 1968, *61,* 817–821.

Pressman, J., & Keleman, G.   Physiology of the larynx. *Physiological Reviews,* 1955, *35,* 506–554.

Ramsey, G., Watson, J., Gramiak, R., & Weinberg, S.   Cinefluoroscopic analysis of the mechanism of swallowing. *Radiology,* 1955, *64,* 498–518.

Richmond, W., Storey, A., & Doty, R.   Integration of deglutition after various transections of medulla oblongata. *Physiologist,* 1960–1961, 3–4, 94.

Robbins, J., Logemann, J., & Kirshner, H.   Velopharyngeal activity during speech and swallowing in neurologic disease. Paper presented at the American Speech-Language-Hearing Association annual meeting, Toronto, 1982.

Roueche, J.   *Dysphagia: An assessment and management program for the adult.* Minneapolis: Sister Kenny Institute, 1980.

Sessle, B., & Hannan, A. (Eds.).   *Mastication and swallowing.* Toronto: University of Toronto Press, 1976.

Sessle, B., & Kenny, D.   Control of tongue and facial motility: Neural mechanisms that may contribute to movements such as swallowing and sucking. *Symposium on Oral Sensation and Perception,* 1973, *4,* 222–231.

Shedd, D., Kirchner, J., & Scatliff, J.   Oral and pharyngeal components of deglutition. *Archives of Surgery,* 1961, *82,* 371–380.

Shedd, D., Scatliff, J., & Kirchner, J.   The buccopharyngeal propulsive mechanism in human deglutition. *Surgery,* 1960, *48,* 846–853.

Shedd, D., Scatliff, J., Chase, R., & Kirchner, J.   Observations on the function of the faucial isthmus in deglutition. *Journal of Surgical Research,* 1961, *1,* 291–300.

Shipp, T., Deatsch, W., & Robertson, K. Pharyngoesophageal muscle activity during swallowing in man. *Laryngoscope,* 1970, *1,* 1–16.

Sloan, R., Ricketts, R., Brummett, S., Bench, R., & Westover, J. L.   Quantified cinefluorographic techniques used in oral roetgenology. *Oral Surgery,* 1965, *20,* 456–462.

Sokol, E., Heitmann, P., Wolf, B., & Cohen, B.   Simultaneous cineradiographic and manometric study of the pharynx, hypopharynx, and cervical esophagus. *Gastroenterology,* 1966, *51,* 960–974.

Sonies, B., Shawker, T., Hall, T., Gerber, L., Whitehouse, W., & Leighton, S.   Ultrasonic visualization of tongue motion during speech. Paper presented at the annual convention of the American Speech Language Hearing Association, Chicago, November 1980.

Spoerel, W.   The unprotected airway. *International Anesthesiology,* 1972, *10,* 1–35.

Stevens, D.   Ultrasound swallow. *British Medical Journal,* 1978, *2,* 1789–1790.

Storey, A.   Interactions of alimentary and upper respiratory tract reflexes. In B. J. Sessle & A. G. Hannan (Eds.), *Mastication and swallowing.* Toronto: University of Toronto Press, 1976.

Sumi, T.   Role of the pontine reticular formation in the neural organization of deglutition. *Japanese Journal of Physiology,* 1972, *22,* 295–314.

Vantrappen, G., & Hellemans, J.   Studies on the normal deglutition complex. *American Journal of Digestive Diseases,* 1967, *12,* 255–266.

Wictorin, W., Hedegard, B., & Lundberg, M.   Cineradiographic studies of bolus position during chewing. *Journal of Prosthetic Dentistry,* 1971, *26,* 236–246.

Wildman, A.   The motor system: A clinical approach. *Dental Clinics of North America,* 1976, *20,* 691–705.

Wright, S.   The radiographic anatomy of patients who gag with dentures. *The Journal of Prosthetic Dentistry,* 1981, *45,* 127–133.

Yotsuya, H., Nonaka, K., & Yoshinobu, I.   Studies on positional relationships of the movements of the pharyngeal organs during deglutition in relation to the cervical vertebrae by X-ray TV cinematography. *Bulletin of the Tokyo Dental College,* 1981, *22,* 159–170.

Yotsuya, H., Saito, Y., & Yoshinobu, I.   Studies on temporal correlations of the movements of the pharyngeal organs during deglutition by X-ray TV cinematography. *Bulletin of the Tokyo Dental College,* 1981, *22,* 171–181.

3

Disorders of Deglutition

Methods of Description

Disorders of deglutition may be described according to symptomatology, clinical or radiographic, and according to the specific abnormalities in anatomy or neuromuscular functioning that result in the disturbed motility patterns seen on X-ray or at the bedside. It is important to differentiate symptoms from anatomic or neuromuscular dysfunctions, as information on the symptoms and dysfunctions is used differently. Symptoms determined clinically and radiographically alert the clinician that the patient's swallowing is disordered, and point toward the nature of the dysfunction. The anatomic and/or neuromuscular dysfunctions are the actual disorders leading to the symptom for which treatment is designed.

Usually, the clinician begins to examine a patient with disordered deglutition by identifying clinical symptoms from careful history taking, chart review, patient descriptions, and a thorough bedside examination. A radiographic study (videofluoroscopy) should then be completed on any patient whose disordered deglutition is not clearly limited to the oral cavity or who may be aspirating. The clinician then uses the information from the videofluoroscopic study to: (1) define anatomic and/or neuromuscular dysfunctions present in the patient's swallow; (2) determine whether the patient should eat by mouth or not, and if so, the consistency of foods to be given, and (3) plan direct or indirect treatment appropriate for the specific swallowing disorders.

This chapter defines the anatomic and neuromuscular disorders, as well as the symptoms of each disorder as might be described by a patient, observed in a bedside clinical evaluation, and observed radiographically. Table 3-1 summarizes symptomology in relationship to the specific anatomic and neuromuscular dysfunctions affecting disorders of mastication, preparation for the swallow, the oral phase of the swallow, the swallowing reflex, the pharyngeal phase of the swallow, and the cervical esophageal phase. Following this organizational format, a clinician may use any or all of the three types of information that might be available to diagnose swallowing dysfunctions.

TABLE 3-1
Clinical and Radiographic Symptoms Corresponding to the Various Neuromuscular and Anatomic Disorders of Swallowing.

Patient Description	Clinical (Bedside) Symptom	Radiographic[2] Symptom	Motility (Neuromuscular) Anatomic Disorder
Cannot chew—avoids foods requiring mastication.	Material remains midline on tongue or falls into sulcus.	Material remains midline on tongue or falls into sulcus.	Inability to lateralize material with tongue.
None[1]	Material falls into sulci.	Material falls into sulci.	Reduced buccal tension.
	Restricted mandibular movement.	Restricted mandibular movement.	Inability to lateralize mandible.
Cannot "line up" teeth.	Cannot align mandible.	Cannot align mandible and maxilla (A-P view).	Inability to align dentition.
Material goes all over mouth. Food catches in mouth.	Material spreads throughout oral cavity.	Loss of bolus control: Material spreads around oral cavity. Material falls over base of tongue into the valleculae or the airway (aspiration *before* the swallow).	Reduced tongue coordination to form bolus (after mastication) Reduced oral sensation.
Coughing, choking *before* the swallow. Food catches in mouth.	Coughing, choking *before* the swallow.		Reduced tongue coordination to hold bolus (for liquids and paste materials).
Food catches in mouth. Slow eating, worse with solids.	Slowed oral transit times	Slowed oral transit times. Reduced tongue elevation. Collection of material on the hard palate.	Reduced tongue elevation.
Slow eating, worse with solids. None[1]	Slowed oral transit times.	Slowed oral transit times.	Reduced anterior to posterior tongue movement.

Slow eating. None[1]	Slowed oral transit times. Repeated pumping tongue motion.	Disorganized anterior to posterior tongue movement. Repeated tongue pumping. Scarred tongue contour.
Slowed oral transit times.	Slowed oral transit times. Collection of material in tongue depression from scarring, worsened with tongue movement.	
Food catches at base of tongue, high in the throat. None[1]	Hesitation of material in the valleculae *prior* to initiation of the swallowing reflex.	Delayed swallowing reflex.
Slowed oral transit times. Delayed elevation of the hyoid bone and thyroid cartilage.		
Food doesn't go down. No hyoid/thyroid elevation. Slowed oral transit times.	Hesitation of material in the valleculae, with potential spill over into pyriform sinus and/or airway. Aspiration *before* swallow. Expectoration of material.	Absent swallowing reflex.
Food coughed up. Coughing/choking.		
Coughing, choking. Expectoration of material *before* the reflex.		
Coughing, choking *after* the reflex.		
Expectoration of material *after* the reflex	Residue of material in the valleculae *after* the swallow. Residue of material in the pyriform sinus after the swallow.	Reduced pharyngeal peristalsis.

None[1] Some patients are unaware of their swallowing disorder, and may not, therefore, describe any particular problem with eating or drinking.

[2] As viewed laterally unless otherwise noted

TABLE 3-1 (Continued)

Patient Description	Clinical (Bedside) Symptom	Radiographic[2] Symptom	Motility (Neuromuscular) Anatomic Disorder
Some food "sticks" high in the throat.		Residue of material on one side of valleculae and one pyriform sinus.	Unilateral pharyngeal paralysis.
Coughing, choking.	Coughing, choking *after* the swallow. Gargley voice quality. Excessive secretions.	Aspiration (spill-over from pyriform sinuses) *after* the swallow. Collection of material in pyriform sinuses. Prominent P-E segment.	Cricopharyngeal dysfunction.
Material catching at bottom of throat. Regurgitation of food. None[1]			
Coughing, choking.	Coughing, choking *after* swallow. Reduced laryngeal (thyroid) elevation.	Aspiration *after* the swallow. Reduced thyroid elevation.	Reduced laryngeal elevation.
	Coughing, choking *during* swallow.	Aspiration *during* the swallow.	Reduced laryngeal adduction.
Hoarseness. None[1]	Hoarseness.	Reduced vocal cord adduction (A-P view).	
Material caught lower in the throat. None[1]		Collection of material in the cervical esophagus after the swallow.	Reduced esophageal peristalsis.

Regurgitation of food. Coughing, choking *after* the swallow.	Regurgitation of food. Coughing, choking *after* swallow.	Collection of material in a side pocket in the pharynx or esophagus.	Esophageal diverticulum.
None¹		Reflux.	
Regurgitation of food, Coughing, choking *after* the swallow.	Regurgitation of food. Coughing, choking *after* the swallow.	Failure of food to pass through the esophagus. Aspiration *after* the swallow from esophageal "overflow."	Partial or total obstruction in pharynx or esophagus.
Coughing, choking *after* the swallow.	Coughing, choking *after* the swallow.	Material passes from esophagus into trachea.	Tracheoesophageal fistula.
Material leaks out hole.	Material leaks out hole onto skin.	Material leaks through skin.	Pharyngocutaneous fistula.

None¹ Some patients are unaware of their swallowing disorder, and may not, therefore, describe any particular problem with eating or drinking.

² As viewed laterally unless otherwise noted.

Neuromuscular and Anatomic Disturbances

The most important step in evaluation and treatment of disorders of deglutition is relating the symptoms observed clinically or radiographically to the actual anatomic or neuromuscular disorder creating the swallowing disturbance. Disorders are described here in the order that might occur in the mastication and deglutition sequence.

Disorders Affecting Mastication

Mastication precedes deglutition. Normal mastication, as described in Chapter 2, requires intact labial and buccal musculature, lingual musculature, mandible, and maxilla.

Reduced Range of Lateral Tongue Movement

For normal mastication to occur, the tongue must collect the material after the mandible has closed and, as the mandible opens, must move the material back on to the teeth. If lingual lateralization is reduced, the patient will be unable to move material onto the teeth. Therefore, normal chewing will be impaired.

Reduced Buccal Tension/ Buccal Scarring

In order for chewed material to remain on the teeth or to fall medially, rather than into the lateral sulcus between cheek and lower alveolus, the buccal musculature (buccinator, masseter, and the internal and external pterygoids), must have normal tone. With less than normal muscle tone, as may occur with facial paralysis or with scarring from facial surgery for head and neck cancer, material may fall into the lateral sulcus during chewing and may be difficult if not impossible for the patient to extricate.

Reduced Range of Lateral
Mandibular Movement

After surgical removal of a portion of the mandible, as in resection for a cancer of the lateral floor of the mouth, the lateral movement of the mandible may be restricted. Because some degree of lateral movement is necessary as a part of the rotary action of the mandible during chewing, normal mastication will be impaired.

Poor Alignment of
Mandible and Maxilla

After surgical resection of a portion of the mandible, as in treatment for head and neck cancer, uneven muscular pull often results in the remaining mandibular segment drifting toward the operated side and out of proper alignment. Even with effort, the patient may not be able to align upper and lower teeth so as to crush material during chewing.

Reduced Range of
Vertical Tongue Movement

During mastication, the tongue normally is elevated somewhat as it rolls food laterally. This tongue elevation helps to keep food on one side or the other during chewing. Without tongue elevation, food will tend to move throughout the mouth in a less controlled fashion.

If tongue control of the bolus is reduced during mastication, some of the material may be aspirated before the patient initiates the swallow. As the patient is attempting to manipulate food in the mouth, some small bits may fall over the base of the tongue, and if bits fail to lodge in the valleculae or pyriform sinuses, these may fall into the open airway. Usually, the swallowing reflex does not trigger in response to such small amounts of material.

Disorders Affecting
the Preparatory Phase
of the Swallow

As detailed in Chapter 2, following mastication, the food is collected into a bolus prior to initiation of the swallow. This stage of deglutition may be called preparation for the swallow, as the patient is pulling the bolus together prior to initiation of oral transit. In the case of liquid or paste swallows, no mastication is required. The material may be retained in a single lump or bolus prior to initiation of transit, or may be moved around in the mouth and reformulated into a bolus before the swallow is initiated.

Reduced Labial Closure

During mastication, preparation to swallow, and the oral and pharyngeal stages of the swallow, labial closure is maintained. If labial closure is incomplete, food or liquid will fall from the mouth.

Reduced Tongue Movement
to Form the Bolus

When material has been masticated, it spreads over a broader area of the oral cavity. Coordinated tongue movement is required to pull material into a cohesive bolus. Insufficient tongue movement at this point in preparation for the swallow can result in material remaining spread throughout the oral cavity. If tongue movement is severely reduced, the lingual struggling movements which occur as the patient attempts to move the material into a cohesive ball, may result in the opposite action of the food or liquid. That is, the struggling may result in further separation of the material throughout the oral cavity. Some of this bolus may collect in the various sulci around the oral cavity, may collect on the roof of the mouth, or may spread so far afield in the oral cavity that the bolus begins to fall over the base of the tongue and into the pharynx prior to any actual initiation of the swallow. Some of this material may fall as far as into the airway. As the airway is not closed at this point because the swallowing reflex has not been triggered, aspiration through the vocal cords may result.

Reduced Range or Coordination
of Tongue Movement
to Hold the Bolus

When liquid or paste materials are placed into the oral cavity, these have already been formed into a cohesive whole. It is necessary for the tongue to maintain the bolus rather than to form it, as with masticated material. If tongue movement and shaping are reduced, the bolus of liquid or paste may flow throughout the oral cavity. This is a great problem with liquids. In fact, in the 1st second of liquid placement in the oral cavity with reduced tongue movement and shaping, a liquid bolus may spread throughout the oral cavity, fall over the base of the tongue and be partially aspirated. This is caused by reduced tongue movement and inability to maintain a preformed bolus in the front of the oral cavity prior to initiation of any swallow. Any aspiration that may occur as the result of reduced tongue movement in the preparation for the swallow has nothing to do with the intactness of the laryngeal mechanism or of the swallowing reflex, as no reflex or swallow was initiated.

Abnormal Hold Position
of the Bolus

The normal hold position of the bolus immediately prior to initiation of the swallow is between the front and central portions of the tongue and the front to midpalate. Occasionally, the bolus will be held in an abnormal, more anterior position against the central incisors as shown in Figure 3-1 and discussed in Chapter 2.

Reduced Oral Sensitivity

If a portion of the oral cavity loses sensation to light touch, material which lodges in the areas of reduced sensitivity may not be felt by the patient. In some cases, material may be lost in the oral cavity and may fall over the base of the tongue and into the airway before any voluntary swallow is initiated.

Disorders in the preparatory phase of the swallowing may result in aspiration of material *before* the swallow. If the patient loses a part of the

FIGURE 3-1
Lateral radiograph of the oral cavity showing a paste bolus held abnormally far forward against the teeth.

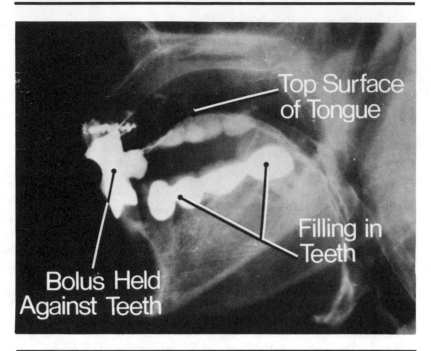

bolus and it falls over the base of the tongue into the pharynx, there is a chance the material will fall into the open airway.

Disorders Affecting
the Oral Phase
of the Swallow

The oral phase of the swallow is defined as the movement of the bolus from the hold position until it passes through the faucial arches. Thus, the timing of the oral phase begins with the first tongue movement to initiate the voluntary aspect of the swallow, and terminates as the bolus passes over the base of the tongue. Normal oral transit time or duration of the oral phase of the swallow is no more than 1 second. A number of motility disorders may occur during the oral phase of the swallow which cause a delay in oral transit.

Tongue Thrust

In tongue thrust, the tongue initiates the swallow with an anterior movement, rather than a coordinated smooth posterior action. The anterior movement is thought to place enough pressure on the central incisors over time to cause them to move anteriorly, out of alignment. In neurologically impaired patients with reduced labial closure, the thrust may push food from the mouth.

Reduced Tongue Elevation

When tongue elevation is restricted because of paralysis or surgical resection, the bolus cannot be moved at the normal speed through the oral cavity. Specifically, with reduced tongue elevation, tongue-to-palate pressures during swallowing are changed and material tends to remain in the front of the mouth, on the tongue, or to collect along the palatal vault, as shown in Figure 3-2. This problem is worst with thick consistency foods. The greater the reduction in tongue elevation, the greater the chance of aspiration. As the patient struggles to move the bolus posteriorly there is increased chance of losing control of the bolus with some of the material falling over the base of the tongue and into the pharynx in small uncontrolled amounts, as shown in Figure 3-3.

Reduced Anterior to Posterior Tongue Movement

In certain types of surgically treated oral cancer patients and neurologically impaired individuals, reduced anterior to posterior tongue movement occurs. Reduction in anterior to posterior movement of the tongue during the swallow slows bolus movement and in many cases causes an increased collection of material in the lateral sulci.

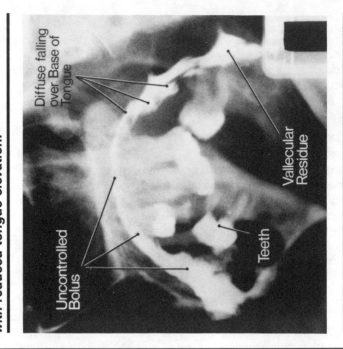

FIGURE 3-3
Lateral radiograph showing the bolus spread from the front of the mouth to the valleculae, as occurs with reduced tongue elevation.

Diffuse falling over Base of Tongue

Vallecular Residue

Uncontrolled Bolus

Teeth

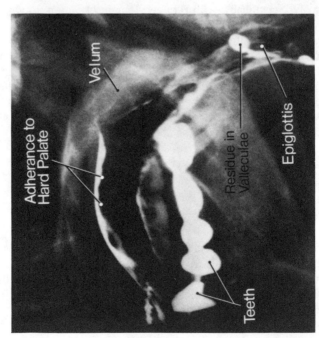

FIGURE 3-2
Lateral radiograph showing a collection of food on the hard palate.

Velum

Adherance to Hard Palate

Residue in Valleculae

Epiglottis

Teeth

Disorganized Anterior to Posterior Tongue Movement

In some neurologically impaired patients, unique patterns of tongue movement may be noted during the oral phase of the swallow. For one example, a repeated pumping action involving both the anterior and posterior tongue may be observed. In this pattern, the bolus is cupped against the palatal vault. As the swallow is initiated, the tongue squeezes the bolus posteriorly but only to the mid palatal region, where the bolus is then rolled forward to its initial position. The swallow may be reinitiated with the squeezing movement of the tongue, but the bolus again reaches the mid to midposterior section of the palate and again rolls anteriorly. The posterior tongue is elevated and remains so during this front to mid-back movement of the bolus. During this time the bolus is not moved over the base of the tongue and the back of the tongue remains elevated. This produces a pumping motion of the front of the tongue with incomplete movement of the bolus through the oral cavity. This is only one example of a disorganized anterior to posterior movement.

Scarred Tongue Contour

After surgical resection of oral carcinoma involving the tongue, scarring of the contour of the tongue may be created. This scarring may result in a depression in the anatomic surface of the tongue, as shown in Figure 3-4. As the tongue moves, a functional depression may be created. That is, as the anterior and posterior sections of the tongue are elevated, the scar tissue being tighter and more bound down, does not elevate to as great an extent as unscarred tissue. Thus, as the tongue is elevated in attempts to swallow, the depression at the point of scarring increases and material collects in it.

Reduced Buccal Tension/ Buccal Scarring

During oral transit reduced buccal tension may result in material falling into the lateral sulcus as the bolus moves posteriorly.

FIGURE 3-4
Lateral radiograph showing collection of barium paste in a depression in the tongue created by scar tissue.

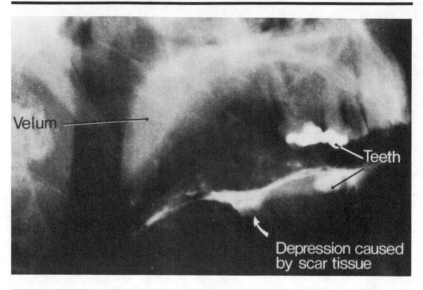

Velum

Teeth

Depression caused by scar tissue

Reduced Ability to Seal Tongue to Palate Laterally

As a result of surgical removal of lateral tongue tissue or unilateral lingual paralysis, the tongue may not seal against the lateral maxillary alveolus on the injured side, resulting in loss of material into the lateral sulcus on that side.

Disorders Affecting the Pharyngeal Phase of the Swallow

When the bolus has reached the faucial arch area at the end of the oral phase of the swallow, the swallowing reflex is normally triggered. When the reflex is triggered, the pharyngeal stage of the swallow begins. The pharyngeal phase of the swallow continues as the bolus is propelled through the pharynx and is terminated as the bolus passes through the P-E segment or the cricopharyngeus muscle. As described in Chapter 2, the pharyngeal phase involves velopharyngeal closure to keep food from entering the nasopharynx, protection of the airway (i.e. complete laryngeal elevation and closure), as well as pharyngeal peristalsis to propel the bolus through the pharynx, and relaxation of the cricopharyngeal musculature to allow the bolus to pass from the pharynx into the esophagus. All of these functions are triggered by the swallowing reflex. Two problems may occur with the swallowing reflex itself.

Delayed Swallowing Reflex

If the swallowing reflex is not triggered as the bolus reaches the faucial arches, the tongue, if normal in function, will compensate by excessive effort to propel the bolus posteriorly so that it falls over the base of the tongue (Kilman & Goyal, 1976). Normally, this bolus falling over the base of the tongue will collect in the valleculae (the area between the base of the tongue and the epiglottis) as shown in Figure 3-5. The bolus may remain there until the reflex is triggered. In some cases this delay in triggering the reflex may be as little as 1 second or may be as long as 5 to 10 seconds or more.

The longer the delay in triggering the reflex, the greater the chance that the patient will aspirate part or all of the bolus. Aspiration can occur during this waiting time because the reflex has not triggered and the airway is open. Any material that has collected in the valleculae may spill over (especially in the case of liquids) and splash or fall into the open airway. This does not reflect an abnormality in laryngeal function, but merely indicates that the reflex has not triggered the larynx to close and protect the airway. If material enters the airway, the cough reflex may be triggered and the patient may expectorate the material. Or, as often occurs in neurologically impaired patients and some surgically treated laryngeal cancer patients, the cough reflex may *not* trigger at all, giving *no* sign of the aspiration. Depending on the viscosity of the material swallowed, it may remain in the valleculae during this delay in reflex triggering, or may spill over and down the aryepiglottic folds into the pyriform sinuses. In some cases, the reflex may not trigger until material reaches the pyriform sinuses. Obviously, the chances of aspiration increase if material must reach the pyriform sinus prior to reflex triggering. If the reflex regularly triggers when material contacts the pyriform sinuses, it is likely the superior laryngeal nerve is responsible for the reflex response rather than the glossopharyngeal nerve.

FIGURE 3-5
Lateral radiograph showing the entire paste bolus resting in the valleculae as can occur when the swallowing reflex does not trigger.

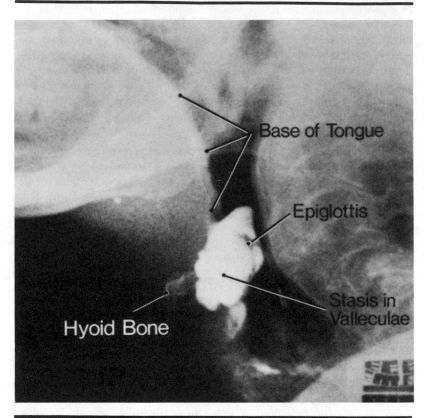

Absent Swallowing Reflex

In some cases, the reflex is not simply delayed, but is entirely absent—no reflex is observed to trigger during the radiographic examination. In these cases, the material may remain in the valleculae while a second and third attempt to swallow occur. At some point the valleculae will fill to overflowing and, if the reflex is entirely absent, this excess material will fall into the airway. In some cases, the valleculae and the pyriform sinuses (the pharyngeal recesses) will fill before the material overflows into the airway. Some patients will cough up or expectorate the entire bolus after it has remained in the valleculae for 10 or more seconds. When the reflex is entirely absent, only two behaviors may result: Either the patient will aspirate the material which collects in the pharynx or he or she will expectorate it.

Inadequate
Velopharyngeal Closure

In patients with partial or total resection of the soft palate, velopharyngeal closure during swallowing may be reduced, allowing some entry of material into the nasal cavity (Edwards, 1976; Kilman & Goyal, 1976). Some neurologically impaired patients exhibit inadequate velopharyngeal closure while others have inaccurate timing of velar movement so that velopharyngeal closure is complete but accomplished too late to completely occlude the velopharyngeal port as the bolus passes, allowing entry of material into the nasal cavity. These problems are usually not severe enough to cause any significant nasal regurgitation. The velopharyngeal gap must be a significant one before the patient will experience large amounts of nasal leakage.

Reduced Pharyngeal
Peristalsis

In many patients with muscular and neuromuscular disorders, as well as those treated for head and neck cancer with radiotherapy or surgical resection including part of the **pharyngeal** wall, pharyngeal peristalsis may be impaired, reducing the squeezing action of the pharyngeal constrictors (Edwards, 1970; Edwards, 1976; Hightower, 1957; Kilman & Goyal, 1976). When this occurs, the entire bolus is not cleared through the pharynx and some residual material is left in the space between the base of the tongue and the epiglottis (the valleculae) and the pyriform sinuses, as shown in Figure 3-6. This disorder is clearly distinguished from a delayed swallowing reflex. With reduced peristalsis, the major part of the bolus moves smoothly through the pharynx with no delay in the triggering of the reflex and no hesitation of the bolus in the valleculae. Rather, *after* the swallow is completed and the pharynx returns to rest, some residue remains in the valleculae and pyriform sinuses. This disorder impairs both sides of the pharyngeal constrictors and is, therefore, distinguished from unilateral paralysis by an equal distribution of residue on both sides of the pharynx. If the residue is excessive, some of the material may fall into the airway *after* the swallow.

FIGURE 3-6
Lateral radiograph showing material left in the valleculae and pyriform sinuses after the swallow.

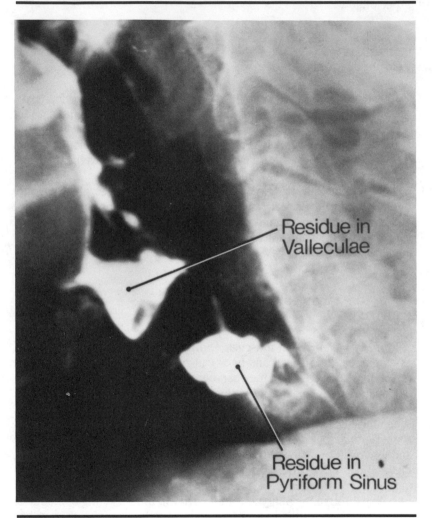

Residue in
Valleculae

Residue in
Pyriform Sinus

**Unilateral Pharyngeal
Paralysis**

When a unilateral pharyngeal paralysis occurs, pharyngeal peristalsis is impaired, including one-half of the cricopharyngeus musculature (High-

FIGURE 3-7
Frontal radiograph showing residue in the pyriform sinuses,
particularly on the right, indicating unilateral pharyngeal
paralysis.

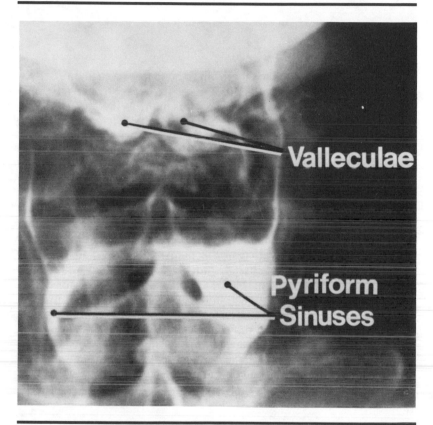

tower, 1957; Kilman & Goyal, 1976). Thus, an A-P radiographic view
shows some residue of material in the valleculae, more on one side than
the other, and a collection of material in the pyriform sinus on the side of
the paralysis as shown in Figure 3-7. Typically, when a patient's head is
tilted toward the *nonparalyzed* side, or when a patient's head is *turned*
toward the *paralyzed* side, material will flow through the normal pyriform
sinus and through the nonparalyzed portion of the cricopharyngeus. Thus,
a unilateral pharyngeal paralysis is distinguished from reduced pharyngeal peristalsis on two bases: (1) the unilateral pharyngeal paralysis
shows symptoms on only one side of the pharynx; and, (2) the unilateral

pharyngeal paralysis involves not only reduced pharyngeal constriction on the side of the paralysis, but also inability of the cricopharyngeus to relax and allow the bolus to pass through the pyriform sinus on the affected side.

Cervical Osteophyte

A cervical osteophyte is an outgrowth of bone from the anterior surface of a cervical vertebra. This anterior bulging narrows the pharynx, sometimes making passage of a normal size bolus difficult (Blumberg, Prapote, & Viscomi, 1977; Gribovsky, 1965; Saunders, 1971). It is rare that the osteophyte is large enough to affect swallowing severely.

Scarred Pharyngeal Wall

Following surgical resection of a portion of the pharyngeal wall or after a pharyngocutaneous fistula has healed, scar tissue in the pharynx may restrict movement of a portion of the pharyngeal constrictors, thereby reducing pharyngeal peristalsis. In some cases, particularly with healed fistula tracts, the scar tissue may form a depression in the pharyngeal wall. This depression will collect material during the swallow, and, at times, may worsen during the swallow as the more mobile portions of the pharynx surrounding the scar tissue constrict with the scar tissue remaining immobile. After the swallow, any food or liquid that remains in the depression created by the scar tissue may be aspirated as the patient opens his or her airway to inhale.

Scar Tissue
at Base of Tongue

In some patients after total laryngectomy, a scar tissue band may form at the base of the tongue, creating a pseudo-epiglottis when viewed laterally. On mirror examination of the pharynx, this scar tissue band, which presents most often after a vertical closure of the surgical wound, may look benign—as if it has little effect on swallowing. However, during attempts at swallowing the contraction of the pharyngeal constrictors will pull the scar tissue band posteriorly, often completely closing off the pharynx and forcing food back into the mouth or up into the nose.

Cricopharyngeal Dysfunction

The cricopharyngeus muscle is in a state of tonic contraction during rest; therefore, as the patient breathes, air is not inhaled into the esophagus simultaneously with inhalation into the lungs. During swallowing, respiration is halted, and the cricopharyngeus must relax as the bolus approaches. If the cricopharyngeus does not relax, or opens too early or too late, the bolus will not pass through the pyriform sinuses and into the esophagus, but will remain in the affected pyriform sinus or sinuses, as shown in Figures 3-8 and 3-9 (Kilman & Goyal, 1976). If this occurs, aspiration may result when material collects in the pyriform sinuses and ultimately overflows into the airway (Calcaterra, Kadell, & Ward, 1975; Harris, 1969; Hawkins, 1967; Parrish, 1968). The mechanism of increased resistance at the cricopharyngeus is not well understood. It has been variably labeled as cricopharyngeal achalasia, functional neuromuscular incoordination, hypopharyngeal bar, and cricopharyngeal spasm. In reality it probably includes several different problems (Cruse, Edwards, Smith, & Wylle, 1979; Kilman & Goyal, 1976; Lund, 1968; Palmer, 1974). Cruse et al. (1979) found changes in the cricopharyngeal muscle in seven patients with dysphagia resulting from obstruction at the cricopharyngeus. This histologic study revealed degeneration and regeneration in muscle fibers with interstitial fibrosis.

Reduced Laryngeal Elevation

During the normal swallow, the larynx is elevated as the tongue is retracted, with the larynx essentially tucked under the base of the tongue (Hightower, 1957). This is one of the mechanisms that effects airway closure and prevents aspiration. If laryngeal elevation is reduced because of paralysis of the strap muscles or surgical resection and reconstruction that interferes with the strap muscles, material will fall to the top of the larynx as it passes through the pharynx, and, unless pharyngeal peristalsis is entirely normal, some material will remain on the top of the airway. After the swallow, when the larynx opens to restore respiration, the residue will fall into the airway.

Reduced Laryngeal Closure

Laryngeal closure to prevent aspiration of material into the trachea *during* the swallow normally occurs at three levels: (1) the epiglottis and

Logemann

FIGURE 3-8
*Lateral radiograph showing liquid in the pyriform sinuses and
the cervical esophagus, with the cricopharyngeal juncture/P-E
segment clearly outlined.*

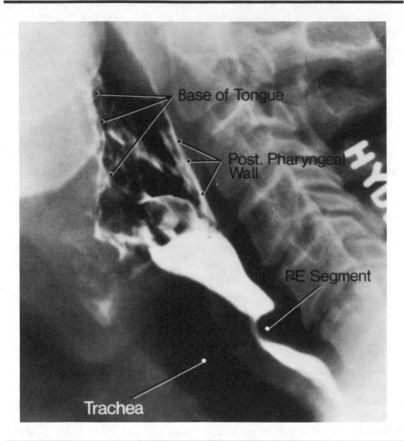

aryepiglottic folds, (2) the false vocal cords and (3) the true vocal cords. If
laryngeal closure is reduced because of neurologic or surgical damage,
airway protection may be compromised so that, while the reflex may be
triggered, material still penetrates the larynx and enters the trachea.
Aspiration due to reduced laryngeal adduction normally occurs as the
bolus is passing through the pharynx. It does not occur as an aftereffect of
the swallow.

FIGURE 3-9
Lateral radiograph showing residue of material in the pyriform sinus with overflow over the arytenoid cartilage and into the airway.

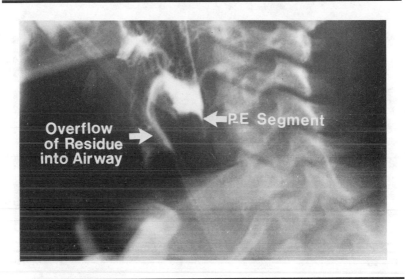

Reduced Laryngeal Closure Resulting from Vocal Cords of Unequal Height

After surgical resection of a portion of the larynx, the remaining tissues on the two sides, particularly the two vocal cords, may be located at unequal height, as shown in Figure 3-10. Thus, though adductor movement of both cords may be normal, the two sides do not complete closure because they do not meet each other. Thus, food can slip between them *during* the swallow.

Postcricoid web

Several authors (Chisholm & Wright, 1967; Cook & May, 1977) have described a postcricoid web arising from the cricoid stretching posteriorly. The web effectively constricts the lower pharynx/upper esophagus, narrowing the lumen. Radiographically, the web appears as a thin

FIGURE 3-10
Frontal radiograph showing the two vocal cords at unequal heights.

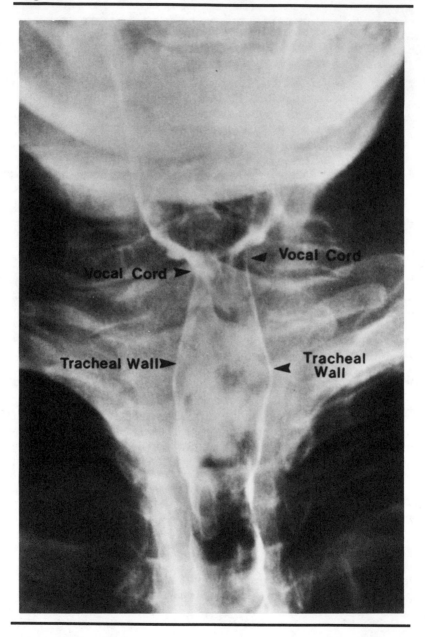

projection from the anterior wall. Several authors (Chisholm & Wright, 1967; Waldenstrom & Kjellberg, 1939) have related the dysphagia to iron deficiency, though others have questioned this relationship (Elwood, Jacobs, Pitman & Entwistle, 1964).

Disorders Affecting the Cervical Esophageal Phase of the Swallow

The cervical esophageal phase of the swallow begins as the bolus passes through the cricopharyngeus musculature and continues until the bolus passes the 7th cervical vertebra. Timing of this phase of the swallow is normally no more than 2 seconds. Several disorders may occur in the cervical esophageal phase of the swallow.

Lax cricopharyngeus

If the cricopharyngeus is too lax, a bolus of material which has entered the cervical esophagus may reflux or return through the cricopharyngeus and into the pharynx. This food may then spill over into the airway.

Reduced Esophageal Peristalsis

Pharyngeal peristalsis or constriction of the pharyngeal constrictors to squeeze the bolus through the pharynx is continued by esophageal musculature to move food through the esophagus. Contraction of this musculature may be reduced as the result of certain neurologic disorders, surgery, or radiotherapy. This reduction will generally result in reduced movement of the bolus and residue of material in the cervical esophagus.

Diverticulum

A diverticulum, or pouch, is a pocket in the pharyngeal and/or esophageal musculature, large enough for a portion or all of the bolus to collect in this side pocket rather than moving smoothly through the pharynx or esophagus (Edwards, 1970; Edwards, 1976). These diverticulae occur most often in the lowest portion of the pharynx or the upper portion of the cervical esophagus and apparently result from a herniation of esophageal musculature. Some authors have suggested diverticula occur as a consequence of pharyngeal dyskinesia and increased pharyngeal pressure due to failure of the cricopharyngeus to relax (Palmer, 1974; Ponzoli, 1968). A diverticulum normally presents radiographically as a ballooning of material that remains in the cervical esophagus after the swallow.

Partial or Total Cervical Esophageal Obstruction

In some cases, the cervical esophagus may stenose or may be blocked by tumor so that material may not pass through (Edwards, 1970; Edwards, 1976; Hawkins, 1967). In these cases, material clearly builds and collects in the cervical esophagus.

Tracheo Esophageal Fistula

A fistula or opening which connects the esophagus to the trachea may occur spontaneously during the healing process after treatment for head and neck cancer, or may result from traumatic injury to the common soft tissue wall between the trachea and the esophagus. In some cases long-term intubation or irritation from a tracheostomy tube (particularly with the cuff inflated) is thought to be the etiologic agent. A tracheo-esophageal fistula allows secretions and food to flow from the esophagus into the trachea.

Esophageal Cutaneous Fistula

Occasionally, after treatment for head and neck cancer, a fistula may form between the esophagus and the external skin, allowing food and saliva to leak out onto the skin.

Aspiration: Review of Etiologies

Aspiration is a generic term referring to the action of material penetrating the larynx and entering the airway below the true vocal folds. One major purpose of any swallowing evaluation is to define the reason for any aspiration present. Once material has entered the airway, it may be expectorated if the patient has an intact cough reflex, plus adequate laryngeal and respiratory control. Or, as is the case with many neurologically impaired patients who have no cough reflex, the material may remain in the trachea and the bronchial tree and be gradually removed by ciliary action. Aspiration pneumonia may result from infiltration of this material into the lungs. If the material swallowed is solid food and has not been masticated well, airway obstruction may result. Because of this possibility for patients who chronically aspirate, it is usually best to feed these patients liquid or paste materials. The amount given per swallow should be restricted to eliminate the possibility of airway obstruction.

The larynx is designed as a three-level valve to protect the airway from entry of food or liquid during swallowing. The valving levels are: (1) the epiglottis and aryepiglottic folds, (2) the false vocal folds, and (3) the true vocal folds. In addition to the three levels of closure of the larynx during swallowing, the elevation of the larynx against the retracted hyoid and base of tongue provides additional protection by essentially tucking the larynx up under the tongue (Kilman & Goyal, 1976).

However as noted in Chapter 2, laryngeal elevation and closure at all three levels of valving in the normal individual occurs during swallowing *only* as a result of the triggering of the swallowing reflex. Airway protection lasts for less than 1 second when the bolus is passing over the base of the tongue.

It is possible to voluntarily protect the airway during swallowing. After removal of the epiglottis and false vocal folds (supraglottic laryngectomy), most patients can successfully relearn to swallow because of the redundancy of laryngeal valving and the availability of voluntary protection measures. In the supraglottic laryngectomy, there is a resection of the top two laryngeal sphincters or airway protectors (i.e. the epiglottis and aryepiglottic folds and the false vocal folds). Postoperatively, patients are taught to protect their airway by closing their remaining sphincter, (the true vocal folds) *voluntarily* during the swallow

For material to be aspirated in the individual with normal anatomy, it must penetrate all three valves of the larynx. This may occur under several circumstances: (1) *before* the swallowing reflex is triggered, when the airway has not elevated or closed; (2) *during* the swallowing if the laryngeal valves are not functioning adequately; and (3) *after* the swallow when the larynx lowers and opens for inhalation.

In order for any of these types of aspiration (before, during or after the swallow) to be treated, it is necessary to identify those defects in oral, pharyngeal, or laryngeal structure or function that cause the particular type of aspiration. Treatment is then directed at the *cause* of the problem, rather than at the result (the aspiration).

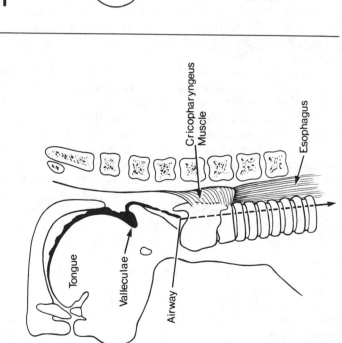

FIGURE 3-12
Aspiration before the swallow because of delayed or absent triggering of the swallowing reflex.

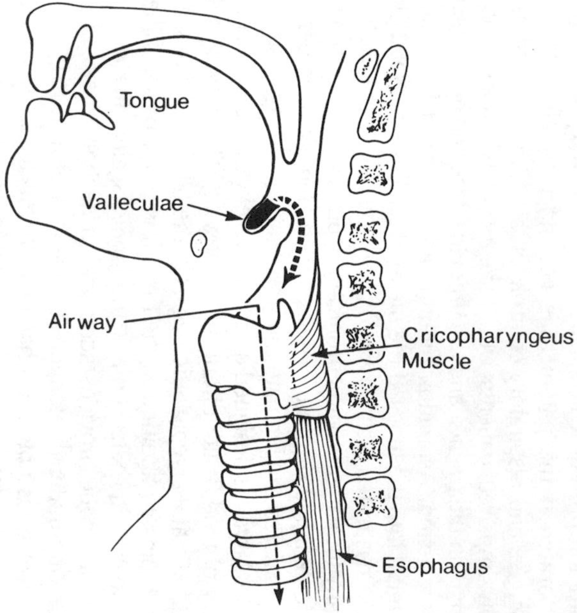

FIGURE 3-11
Aspiration before the swallow because of reduced tongue movement.

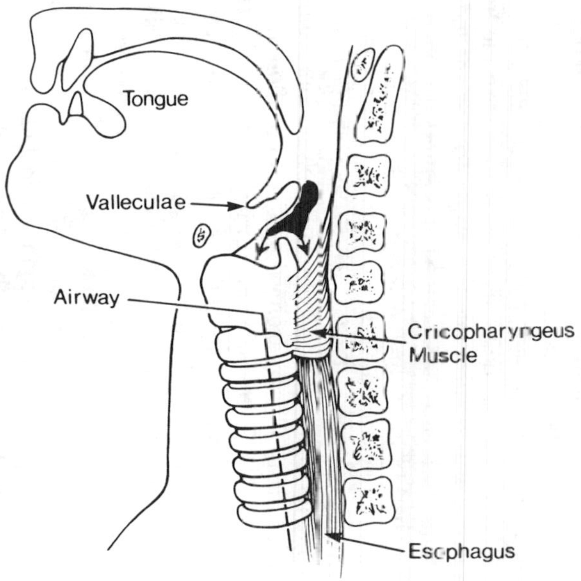

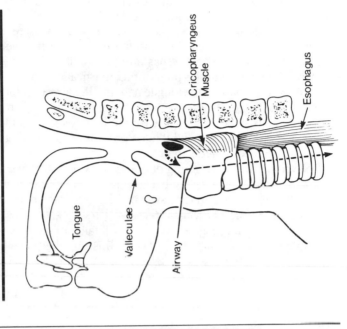

FIGURE 3-14
Aspiration after the swallow when material left in the pyriform sinuses overflows into the airway.

FIGURE 3-13
Aspiration during the swallow because of reduced laryngeal closure.

Aspiration *before* the swallow, as illustrated in Figure 3-11, generally occurs because of reduced tongue control during the oral phase of the swallow, or because of a delayed or absent swallowing reflex. If lingual control is poor, liquid may flow into the mouth and fall over the base of the tongue before the patient has an opportunity to initiate a voluntary swallow. If tongue control is poor during mastication, small pieces of food may fall over the base of the tongue and into the airway before a voluntary swallow is initiated. Patients with poor tongue control often do best with thin paste consistencies that are easier to hold together in the mouth and which do not require forceful tongue propulsion. Treatment involves exercises to improve tongue control.

Delayed or absent triggering of the swallowing reflex will also result in aspiration *before* the swallow because material will be pushed over the base of the tongue but no reflex will be triggered. Material will then either fall into one of the pharyngeal recesses (the valleculae or the pyriform sinuses), as shown in Figure 3-12, or it will fall into the airway. It must be remembered that the airway is open at this time because the reflex has not triggered. Patients with a delayed or absent reflex will usually have greatest difficulty with liquids, since the thinner consistency of material will splash into the pharynx and more often into the airway, whereas thicker consistencies are more apt to slide over the base of the tongue and rest in the valleculae. The reflex does not trigger differently during attempts to swallow the two materials; rather, the variation in viscosity of the two materials results in differences in stability of materials in the pharynx. Aspiration resulting from a delayed or absent reflex is treated by stimulating the swallowing reflex.

Aspiration *during* the swallow occurs because the three sphincters of the larynx fail to close tightly enough to prevent food penetration, as illustrated in Figure 3-13. As the bolus enters the pharynx and passes the larynx, part or all of the bolus enters the airway, while the remainder of the bolus may continue into the esophagus (Kilman & Goyal, 1976). On fluoroscopy some or all of the bolus is seen sliding directly into the airway, meeting no obstruction. Treatment involves improving adduction of the laryngeal tissues by an exercise program or teflon injection.

Aspiration after the swallow can be caused by inadequate pharyngeal peristalsis or hypertonicity of the cricopharyngeus muscle (Palmer, 1974), as shown in Figure 3-14. In either case, the aspiration results from material remaining in pharyngeal recesses *after* the swallow and falling or being sucked into the airway when the larynx lowers and opens after the swallow is completed (Kilman & Goyal, 1976). In the case of reduced pharyngeal peristalsis, the main portion of the bolus moves through the pharynx, but because the strength of peristalsis is reduced, some material is left behind to coat the pharyngeal walls, valleculae, and pyriform sinuses. The larger the amount of residue, the greater the chance of aspiration after the swallow. No treatment currently available will improve pharyngeal peristalsis, though several compensatory techniques are described in Chapter 5.

With a dysfunctioning cricopharyngeus, material cannot enter the esophagus and remains in the pharynx, filling the pyriform sinuses. With each swallow, more and more material will collect in the pharynx, finally overflowing into the airway between swallows. The most frequent treatment for this disorder is cricopharyngeal myotomy.

Each of these five causes of aspiration requires a different treatment. Thus, a major goal of any swallowing evaluation is not only to determine that aspiration occurs, but to identify the *etiology* of the aspiration so that appropriate treatment can be initiated.

Patient Descriptions
of Swallowing Disorders

Clinical symptoms of swallowing disorders are frequently noted by the patient as well as the swallowing therapist. For example, when asked to describe their swallowing problem, patients may complain of coughing or choking, or may describe the feeling of food "catching in their throat" (Phillips & Hendrix, 1971).

During the radiographic studies of swallowing disorders in 1,000 patients at Northwestern University, 750 of whom complained of a variety of swallowing problems, the correlation between the patient's perception of the location and the nature of the disorder and the anatomic location of the actual motility disorders was studied. In all cases when patients described a problem with their eating or swallowing, they were entirely accurate in localizing the problem, though not in identifying the nature of the problem. Specifically, reports of inability to chew were confirmed as one of several disorders affecting mastication. When patients complained of food collecting in the mouth that they were unable to swallow, radiographic studies revealed food remaining in the oral cavity after the attempt to swallow.

Patients describing problems in holding food together in the mouth were confirmed to have difficulty controlling the bolus. If patients described a hesitation and collection of food high in the throat, pointing to the base of the tongue, the disorder observed radiographically was: (1) hesitation of material in the valleculae between the base of the tongue and the epiglottis as a result of a delayed swallowing reflex or (b) residue in the valleculae after the swallow, indicating reduced peristalsis. Patients complaining of choking and coughing *before* starting to swallow were seen to have aspiration before the swallow was initiated, as a result of reduced lingual control or a delayed or absent swallowing reflex. When patients complained of coughing or choking *during* the swallow, some degree of aspiration was always observed *during* the swallow, indicating reduced laryngeal airway protection. When a patient reported coughing after the swallow, they were observed to aspirate after the swallow because of residue in the pharynx resulting from reduced pharyngeal peristalsis, reduced laryngeal elevation, or a dysfunction of the crico-pharyngeus muscle. When patients described a collection of food low in the throat, the radiographic disorder observed was hesitation of material in the cervical esophagus or collection of material in the pyriform sinus, both of which are located in the lower neck region. In some cases, the severity of the disorder was not as great as the patient had described, but the general anatomic localization of symptoms seen radiographically and the patient's localization of the problem did correspond in 99.2% of the cases.

Thus, when a patient describes a swallowing disorder, his or her information should be carefully recorded, as it may point the clinician to the general anatomic area of the dysfunction. Table 3-1 presents the symptoms reported by the 1,000 patients as related to the symptoms observed on clinical examination of the patient, the radiographic symptoms, and the actual anatomic or neuromuscular disorders.

If a patient denies a swallowing disorder, the reports may be highly inaccurate. Of the 250 patients in this group who denied having a swallowing disorder but whose care providers or family identified a difficulty, *all* exhibited abnormal swallowing. This lack of awareness is particularly prevalent in neurologically impaired patients, e.g. those with CVA, Parkinsonism, and multiple sclerosis.

Clinical Bedside Observations

Symptoms which may be observed during a bedside clinical examination of swallowing are generally rather gross and do not provide enough detailed information to permit identification of the specific anatomic or neuromuscular problem causing the symptom. However, clinical symptoms can identify the area of dysfunction, i.e. the oral stage versus pharyngeal stage of the swallow.

Beginning in the oral cavity with the preparatory phase of the swallow, the following symptoms may be noted in a bedside swallowing evaluation.

1. *Pocketing of food in the lateral sulcus,* observed by asking the patient to open his or her mouth after the swallow, is a symptom of reduced buccal tension because of neurologic or anatomic damage. Normally, as the bolus is pushed backward when the swallow is initiated, the bolus remains a cohesive mass and does not fall into the sulci between the cheek and lower alveolis.

2. *Collection of food in the anterior sulcus or beneath the tongue anteriorly or laterally,* also observed by asking the patient to open his or her mouth after the swallow, results from reduced tongue function because of neurologic damage or surgical resection.

3. *Collection of food on the hard palate,* observed after the swallow when the patient opens his or her mouth, indicates reduced tongue elevation. Normally, the tongue sweeps material posteriorly along the hard palate, cleaning it at the same time. If range of tongue elevation is reduced, the material may adhere to the palate and remain there after the attempt to swallow.

4. *Spitting food out of the mouth,* when the swallow is initiated may indicate a tongue thrusting behavior in the oral phase of the swallow. This thrusting behavior, or forward movement of the tongue to initiate the swallow rather than normal upward and backward tongue movement, can cause materials to fall from the mouth, particularly if labial closure is poor. In some instances, obviously, uncooperative adults and children may voluntarily spit food from the mouth. Food falling from the mouth may also indicate reduced labial closure with normal tongue movement. If the material is coughed from the mouth several seconds or more after the swallow is initiated it may indicate an absent swallowing reflex.

5. *Slowed oral transit times* result from any abnormality in swallowing in the oral phase of the swallow. Thus, the slowed times, whether measured at bedside or radiographically, indicate a problem in the oral phase of the swallow, which must be defined. Techniques for measuring oral transit at the bedside are described in Chapter 4.

6. *Excessive lingual movement* may be felt by placing a finger under the mandible as the patient attempts to swallow. This excessive movement may reflect discoordinated tongue gestures as the

patient attempts to propel the bolus or may indicate the patient's attempt to compensate for a delayed or absent swallowing reflex by pushing material into the pharynx with the tongue (as described earlier).

7. *Delayed or absent elevation of the hyoid bone and thyroid cartilage,* observed by placing one finger on the hyoid and one on the thyroid as the patient swallows, indicates a late or totally absent swallowing reflex. A major consequence of the reflex triggering is the elevation (and closure) of the larynx to protect the airway. If the patient compensates for a late reflex by increasing tongue activity, the hyoid bone will move a great deal. This movement may mislead the clinician into thinking the reflex has triggered.

8. *Coughing and choking* before, during, or after the reflexive swallow usually indicates aspiration or entry of material into the airway. The cough reflex normally triggers if material enters the larynx and touches the false or true vocal cords. Normally, the larynx is elevated and closed tightly during deglutition, preventing aspiration. However, if oral control of the bolus is poor, with material falling into the pharynx *prior to initiation of the swallow,* or if the larynx does not close tightly enough *during the swallow,* of if any amount of food is left in the pharynx *after the swallow,* this material may fall into the airway and cause the patient to cough and choke. It should always be remembered, however, that many patients have aspiration, or entry of material into the airway, without eliciting any cough reflex. These silent aspirators make careful radiographic evaluation of the motility patterns of deglutition essential.

9. *A gargly voice quality* on vocalization after a swallow may also indicate aspiration. In the normal swallow, material does not contact the true vocal cords, and following the swallow, no material is left in the larynx. If material does enter the larynx before, during, or after the swallow it may remain there when the patient attempts to phonate and cause a very gargly, wet vocal quality.

10. *Excessive, copious secretions* are also a symptom of aspiration. These secretions may appear to consist of saliva and mucous with no trace of food substance. However, these secretions generally indicate an attempt of the cilia in the respiratory tract to clear away foreign material. Excessive and copious secretions are a very obvious symptom of aspiration but may sometimes be misidentified as symptoms of allergy or infection. Often, this patient will have no fever concurrent with these excessive secretions. Patients often describe the problem as excessive saliva and mucous.

11. *Expectoration or regurgitation of material through the mouth or nose* may be the result of a pharyngeal or esophageal obstruction or may be the patient's way of getting rid of material from the pharynx when the swallowing reflex does not trigger. Similarly, if a pharyngeal or esophageal diverticulum empties, the material might be regurgitated or expectorated. Material passing through a tracheoesophageal fistula will also be expectorated, as will most material which is aspirated. Material which is coughed or regurgitated may exit the nose if the soft palate is lowered. Since this coughing or regurgitation occurs *after* the swallowing reflex has triggered, when the soft palate (velum) is normally lowered and the velopharyngeal port is open, food or liquid is free to enter the nose. Thus, this nasal regurgitation *usually* does not indicate velopharyngeal incompetence or malfunction.

Table 3-1 relates these clinical symptoms to patient descriptions, radiographic symptoms, and anatomic and neuromuscular disorders.

Radiographic Symptoms—
Lateral Plane

Radiographic symptoms of disorders of deglutition are described here as observed on lateral and anterior/posterior fluoroscopic views. The procedure for the videofluoroscopic study is described in Chapter 4.

The following radiographic symptoms are observed on lateral fluoroscopy. Additional symptoms that can be noted in the A-P view are described at the end of this chapter.

Preparation to Swallow

Material Remains at Midline
or Falls into the Sulci

If mastication is necessary prior to deglutition, the bolus is normally moved laterally in a rotary fashion by the tongue. If lateral tongue movement is not present, vertical tongue movement may be used to mash the food. Otherwise, food will remain on the tongue or fall between tongue and teeth.

Limited Mandibular Movement

Normal mandibular movement for mastication is rotary. If lateral mandibular movement is not possible, only vertical movement will be observed on attempts to chew.

Loss of Bolus Control

One of the first symptoms which may be seen when food is placed in the mouth is a loss of control of the bolus in the oral cavity before the swallow is initiated. The material (liquid, paste) spreads throughout the oral cavity and is not maintained in a cohesive mass by the tongue prior to the swallow. Normally, in preparation for the swallow after mastication has occurred, i.e. immediately prior to initiation of swallowing, the bolus should be brought together from around the mouth into a cohesive ball for propulsion by the tongue. Material should not fall over the base of the tongue in bits and pieces prior to initiation of the swallow.

Oral Stage of the Swallow

Slowed Oral Transit Time

Once the backward lingual propulsion of the bolus has begun, oral transit time should be no more than 1 second. Oral transit time is defined as the time taken from the initiation of the swallow until the bolus passes through the faucial arches. Slowed oral transit time (time greater than 1 second) indicates a motility problem in the oral phase of the swallow.

Stasis in Anterior Sulcus

Material will collect in the space between the anterior portion of the alveolar ridge and the lower lip if anterior lingual control is poor or if there is a surgical defect anteriorly.

Stasis in the Lateral Sulcus

Collection of material between the lateral alveolar ridge and the cheek results when the normal muscle tone in the cheek is disturbed.

Stasis in Mid-Tongue Depression

Collection of material in a depression in the tongue usually worsens as the patient attempts to clear the material by elevating the surrounding tongue. This collection of material indicates scar tissue on the tongue.

Stasis on the Tongue

If tongue movement is severely reduced, material remains on the tongue. Generally, food must be of a thick consistency to stay on the tongue and not fall onto the floor of the mouth.

Incomplete Tongue to Palate Contact

Reduced tongue elevation and contact to the palate may be observed in the oral phase of the swallow. This results in a residue of material on the hard palate after the swallow or in material staying on the tongue, as described above.

Disturbed Lingual Peristalsis

Instead of the normal organized, smooth anterior to posterior movement of the tongue to propel the bolus posteriorly, there may be an irregular struggle activity or a regular repetitive pattern, such as a rolling backward and forward. There may be a number of distinct patterns included in this disorder, some of which are characteristic of particular disease entities, such as Parkinsonism, as described in Chapter 8.

Adherence to Hard Palate

In addition to slowed oral transit times, reduced tongue control can be indicated by material pooling or adhering to structures in the oral cavity.

This residue of material adheres to the hard palate after the swallow is completed. This typically worsens with materials of thicker consistency and in some cases the majority of the bolus remains on the palate. The bolus divides and only part proceeds on into the pharynx and the pharyngeal stage of the swallow.

Reduced Anterior/Posterior Tongue Movement

During the oral phase of the swallow, the range of anterior to posterior tongue movement may be reduced so the tongue does not move as far posteriorly as normal during the propulsion of the bolus.

Uncontrolled Bolus/ Premature Swallow

If a part of the bolus is lost because of reduced tongue control, it may fall over the base of the tongue prematurely before the voluntary swallow is initiated. This material will fall into the pharynx and if not caught in the valleculae, may fall into the open airway.

Piecemeal Deglutition

Rather than swallowing the entire bolus at one time, piecemeal deglutition refers to division of the bolus into two or three swallows. If a large amount of material is put into the mouth at one time, piecemeal deglutition is normal. However, if a bolus consists of ⅓ to ½ a teaspoon of material, a single swallow should be all that is needed to clear material from the oral cavity.

Late or Insufficient Velar Elevation

The velum normally elevates as the bolus reaches the faucial arches and triggers the swallowing reflex. The velum remains elevated only until the bolus passes the oropharynx. Occasionally, velar elevation may be late or insufficient to complete velopharyngeal closure, so some food is seen to enter the nasal cavity.

Pharyngeal Stage
of the Swallow

Slowed Pharyngeal
Transit Time

A major radiographic symptom of pharyngeal disorders is slowed pharyngeal transit time. Pharyngeal transit time is defined as the time it takes for the bolus to pass from the faucial arches over the base of the tongue and through the pyriform sinus into the esophagus. Normally, pharyngeal transit time should be no more than 1 second. If pharyngeal transit time is increased, motility problems are present and must be identified.

Scar Tissue at
Base of Tongue

A scar tissue band can be easily viewed as extra tissue which forms a pocket at the base of the tongue where food collects.

Vallecular Stasis:
Hesitation of Material
in the Valleculae Prior
to Initiation of
the Swallowing Reflex

Material may fall over the base of the tongue and into the valleculae where it hesitates for several seconds or more before the swallowing reflex is triggered. This hesitation of the bolus indicates a late swallowing reflex. Depending on the viscosity of the material swallowed, it may splash from the valleculae onto the aryepiglottic folds and into the airway, where the material is aspirated before the swallowing reflex is triggered. If the reflex does not trigger for 30 seconds, it should be declared absent.

Cervical Osteophyte

Radiographically, a cervical osteophyte can be seen as a boney outgrowth, or protrusion, from one or more of the cervical vertebrae. If large enough, an osteophyte may impinge on the pharynx and narrow it so food, particularly of thicker consistency, cannot pass easily.

Coating of Pharyngeal Walls After the Swallow

Another symptom of reduced pharyngeal peristalsis is a residue of barium on the pharyngeal walls, coating the tissue and remaining after the swallow.

Residue of Material in the Valleculae after the Triggering of the Swallowing Reflex

Although the swallowing reflex triggers on time and the bolus does not hesitate in the valleculae, a residue of material may remain in the valleculae after the swallow. This residue generally indicates a reduction in the strength of pharyngeal peristalsis. Residue on only one side generally indicates a weakness on that side of the pharynx.

Collection of Material in a Pharyngeal Depression

If scar tissue is present in the pharynx, it often creates a depression in the soft tissues of the pharyngeal wall. As the bolus passes through the pharynx, some of the material may collect in this depression and remain after the swallow.

Reduced Thyroid Elevation

Normally, the thyroid cartilage should elevate simultaneously with the triggering of the swallowing reflex to assist in closing the airway. If elevation is late or reduced, food will be seen to rest on the top of the larynx in the laryngeal vestibule and may be seen to enter the airway after the swallow when the patient opens his or her airway to inhale.

Reduced Laryngeal Closure

If the larynx does not close during the swallow, aspiration is seen *during* the swallow, so that a part or all of the bolus enters the airway with no hesitation.

Collection of Material in
One or Both Pyriform Sinuses

Normally, the bolus divides and passes through the two pyriform sinuses and through the cricopharyngeus muscle or pharyngo-esophageal segment (P-E segment) into the esophagus. If the P-E segment does not relax easily to allow food to pass, material will collect in the pyriform sinuses and may overflow after several swallows into the airway, causing aspiration. If only one side of the P-E segment or pharynx is affected, material will collect in only one pyriform sinus.

Aspiration

Another disorder in the pharyngeal stage of the swallow observed radiographically is *aspiration,* or entry of material into the trachea. Aspiration does not always coincide with increased pharyngeal transit time, though it may. Aspiration can be seen when the larynx does not close normally *during* the swallow. However, aspiration can also be observed *before* the swallow because of poor tongue control or a delayed or absent swallowing reflex, or *after* the swallow because residual material in the pharynx falls into the airway.

Radiographic Symptoms—
Anterior-Posterior Plane

Six important radiographic observations can be made in the anterior-posterior plane: alignment of the mandible, symmetry of pooling in oral cavity, degree of vocal cord adduction, equal height of vocal cords, symmetry of vallecular stasis, and the symmetry of stasis in the pyriform sinuses.

TABLE 3-2
Data Collection Sheet for Fluoroscopic Studies of Deglutition.

Northwestern University
FLUOROSCOPIC EXAMINATION OF SWALLOWING
Jeri A. Logemann, PhD

Patient's name _____ Age _____

Date of study _____ Date oral feeding began _____

Etiology of patient's swallowing disorder _____

Purpose of study _____

Timing and motility disorders	Liquid	Paste[1]	Masticated Material	Swallowing Disturbances
Preparation to swallow:				
Mastication:				
Unable to align teeth	---	---	---	
Unable to lateralize material	---	---	---	Reduced tongue lateralization
Unable to mash material	---	---	---	
Bolus formation:				
Cannot hold food in mouth	---	---	---	Reduced lip closure
Cannot form bolus	---	---	---	Reduced range or coordination of tongue movement
Cannot hold bolus	---	---	---	
Other _____	---	---	---	

Oral transit time:

Stasis in anterior sulcus	——— ——— ———	Reduced buccal tension
Stasis in lateral sulcus	——— ——— ———	*Tongue scarring
Stasis in mid-tongue depression	——— ——— ———	
Stasis on tongue	——— ——— ———	
Disturbed lingual peristalsis	——— ——— ———	Disorganized anterior to posterior tongue movement
Incomplete tongue to palate contact	——— ——— ———	Reduced tongue elevation
Adherence to hard palate	——— ——— ———	
Reduced anterior/posterior tongue movement	——— ——— ———	Reduced anterior/posterior tongue movement
Uncontrolled bolus/premature swallow	——— ——— ———	
Aspiration (%) *before* swallow	——— ——— ———	
Piecemeal deglutition	——— ——— ———	
Late velar elevation	——— ——— ———	
Other _____	——— ——— ———	

---

[1]Space provided for data on 3 swallows per consistency.
*Anatomic problems

TABLE 3-2 (Continued)

Timing and motility disorders	Liquid	Paste[1]	Masticated Material	Swallowing Disturbances
Pharyngeal transit time:				
Diffuse falling over base of tongue	— — —	— — —	— — —	*Scar tissue—base of tongue
Scar tissue-base of tongue	— — —	— — —	— — —	Delayed reflex
Late swallowing reflex-vallecular stasis	— — —	— — —	— — —	Absent reflex
Absent swallowing reflex	— — —	— — —	— — —	
Aspiration (%) *before swallow*	— — —	— — —	— — —	*Cervical osteophyte
Cervical osteophyte	— — —	— — —	— — —	Reduced peristalsis
Coating of pharyngeal walls after swallow	— — —	— — —	— — —	
Vallecular residue (%) after swallow	— — —	— — —	— — —	
Aspiration (%) *after swallow*	— — —	— — —	— — —	*Scar tissue—pharyngeal wall
Scar tissue—pharyngeal wall	— — —	— — —	— — —	Reduced laryngeal elevation
Reduced laryngeal elevation	— — —	— — —	— — —	
Aspiration (%) *after swallow*	— — —	— — —	— — —	Reduced laryngeal closure
Reduced laryngeal closure	— — —	— — —	— — —	
Aspiration (%) *during swallow*	— — —	— — —	— — —	Cricopharyngeal dysfunction
Stasis/residue in both pyriform sinuses	— — —	— — —	— — —	Pharyngeal hemiparesis
Residue in one pyriform sinus right—left	— — —	— — —	— — —	
Aspiration (%) *after swallow*	— — —	— — —	— — —	
Cervical esophageal stage:				
Esophageal/pharyngeal reflux	— — —	— — —	— — —	Cricopharyngeal dysfunction
Tracheo-esophageal fistula	— — —	— — —	— — —	*T-E fistula
Zenker's diverticulum	— — —	— — —	— — —	*Zenker's diverticulum

[1]Space provided for data on 3 swallows per consistency.
*Anatomic problems

Oral Stage
of the Swallow

Misaligned Mandible

Alignment of mandibular and maxillary teeth can be easily examined in an A-P view of the oral cavity during fluoroscopy.

Symmetry of Pooling
in Oral Cavity

With the patient turned anteriorly, the location of residual material on each side of the oral cavity can be clearly seen.

Pharyngeal Stage
of the Swallow

Reduced Vocal Cord Adduction

An A-P view of the trachea with the patient's head extended permits examination of vocal cord movements, specifically the symmetrical nature of the movement during phonation and deglutition.

Unequal Height of
the Vocal Cords

Viewing the larynx anteriorly as the patient tilts his head back reveals the relative height of the two vocal cords so that any difference in height can be easily observed.

Asymmetrical
Vallecular Stasis

An A-P view of the base of the tongue reveals the collection of material on either side of the valleculae.

Asymmetrical Stasis
in the Pyriform Sinuses

Collection of material in the pyriform sinuses may be unilateral or bilateral. An A-P view reveals any asymmetries in this stasis.

When initially examining videofluoroscopic studies of deglutition, it is sometimes helpful to have a check sheet to catalog behaviors observed. Table 3-2 presents one example of a data collection sheet for use in structuring radiographic observations.

Bibliography

Blumberg, P., Prapote, C., & Viscomi, G.   Cervical osteophytes producing dysphagia. *Ear, Nose and Throat Journal,* 1977, *56,* 15–21.

Calcaterra, T., Kadell, B., & Ward, O.   Dysphagia secondary to cricopharyngeal muscle dysfunction. *Archives of Otolaryngology,* 1975, *101,* 726–729.

Castell, D., Knuff, T., Brown, F., Gerhardt, D., Burns, T., & Gaskins, R.   Dysphagia. *Gastroenterology,* 1979, *76,* 1015–1024.

Chisholm, M., & Wright, R.   Postcricoid dysphagia and iron deficiency in men. *British Medical Journal,* 1967, *2,* 281–283.

Cohen, S.   Difficulty in swallowing as an early sign. *Clinical Pediatrics,* 1971, *10,* 682.

Cook, P., & May, B.   A posterior pharyngeal web in sideropenic dysphagia. *Journal of Laryngology and Otology,* 1977, *91,* 989–992.

Cruse, J., Edwards D., Smith, J., & Wylle, J.   The pathology of a cricopharyngeal dysphagic. *Histopathology,* 1979, *3,* 223–232.

Donald A., & Dawes, J.   A case of dysphagia. *British Medical Journal,* 1977, *1,* 1139–1141.

Edwards D.   Flow charts, diagnostic keys and algorithms in the diagnosis of dysphagia. *Scottish Medical Journal,* 1970, *15,* 378–385.

Edwards, D.   The problem of dysphagia. *Practitioner,* 1976, *216,* 631–636.

Elwood, P., Jacobs, A., Pitman, R., & Entwistle, C.   Epidemiology of the Paterson-Kelly Syndrome, Lancet, 1964, *2,* 716–720.

Gribovsky, E.   Dysphagia in association with hyperexostoses of the cervical vertebrae. *American Journal of Gastroenterology,* 1965, *45,* 284–286.

Haider, Z., & Kaiamchi, S.   Painful dysphagia due to fracture of the styloid process. *Oral Surgery, Oral Medicine and Oral Pathology,* 1980, *49,* 5–6.

Harris, L. Dysphagia. *Advances in Internal Medicine,* 1969, *15,* 203–219.

Hawkins, C. Dysphagia. Diseases of the digestive system. *British Medical Journal,* 1967, *4,* 663–667.

Henderson, R., Woolf, C., & Marryatt, G. Pharyngoesophageal dysphagia and gastroesophageal reflux. *Laryngoscope, 86,* 1976, 1531–1539.

Hightower, N. Newer concepts of the physiology of deglutition and dysphagia, *American Journal of Surgery,* 1957, *93,* 154–162.

Hurwitz, M. Taking a good look at the problem of dysphagia. *Geriatrics,* 1973, *28,* 50–55.

Kilman, W., & Goyal, R. Disorders of pharyngeal and upper esophageal sphincter motor function. *Archives of Internal Medicine,* 1976, *136,* 592–601.

Kumpe, D. Dysphagia for several years. *Journal of the American Medical Association,* 1971, *216,* 116–117.

Lund, W. The cricopharyngeal sphincter: Its relationship to the relief of pharyngeal paralysis and the surgical treatment of the early pharyngeal pouch. *Journal of Laryngology and Otology,* 1968, *82,* 353–367.

McHardy, G. Dysphagic problems. *Postgraduate Medicine,* 1968, *44,* 125–127.

Nelson, P. Observations on dysphagia. *Medical Journal of Australia,* 1970, *2,* 924–930.

Palmer, E. Dysphagia due to cricopharyngeus dysfunction. *American Family Physician,* 1974, *9,* 127–131.

Park. D. Dysphagia. *British Medical Journal,* 1977, *1,* 977.

Parrish, R. Cricopharyngeus dysfunction and acute dysphagia, *Canadian Medical Association Journal,* 1968, *99,* 1167–1171

Phillips, M., & Hendrix, T. Dysphagia. *Postgraduate Medicine,* 1971, *50,* 81–86.

Pitcher, J. Dysphagia in the elderly: causes and diagnosis. *Geriatrics,* 1973, *28,* 64–69.

Ponzoli, V. Zenker's diverticulum: A review of pathogeneses and presentation of 25 cases. *Southern Medical Journal,* 1968, *61,* 817–821.

Press, H. D., & Leffall, L. D. Hoarseness and dysphagia secondary to cervical hyperostosis. Report of an unusual case. *Medical Annals of the District of Columbia,* 1972, *41,* 26–28.

Pullen, I. A case of dysphagia. *British Medical Journal,* 1977, *1,* 1353.

Saunders, W. Cervical osteophytes and dysphagia. *Journal of Otology, Physiology and Laryngology,* 1971, *79,* 1091–1097.

Schultz, A. R., Niemtzow, P., Jacobs, S. R., & Naso, F. Dysphagia associated with cricopharyngeal dysfunction. *Archives of Physical Medicine and Rehabilitation,* 1979, *60,* 381–386.

Waldenstrom, J., & Kjellberg, S. Roentgenologic diagnosis of sidero-penic dysphagia (Plummer-Vinson syndrome), *Acta Radiologica*, 1939, *20*, 618–638.

Walker, J. A., & Rogers, A. I. Dysphagia. *Postgraduate Medicine*, 1978, *64*, 159–164.

4

Evaluation of Swallowing Disorders

This chapter reviews two procedures for the evaluation of patients with swallowing disorders: (1) the videofluoroscopic study known as the modified barium swallow or "cookie swallow," and (2) the bedside or clinical examination.

Videofluoroscopic Procedure

Because swallowing is a dynamic and rapid process, fluoroscopy is particularly well suited to the study of this physiologic function (Dobie, 1978; Kirchner, 1967; Linden & Siebens, 1980; O'Connor & Ardran, 1976; Pitcher, 1973; Sloan, 1977).

How the fluoroscopic image is recorded for permanent storage may vary from one institution to another. *Cine*fluoroscopy or the recording of the fluoroscopic image on movie film, has the advantage of permitting frame-by-frame analysis of the movement patterns of various structures and of the bolus of food or liquid (Kelley, 1970; Phillips & Hendrix, 1971; Schultz, Niemtzow, Jacobs, & Naso, 1979; Sloan et al. 1977). However, radiation exposure during cinefluoroscopy is greater than the alternative method of recording, i.e. videofluoroscopy, and is becoming less available in the average hospital. Also, no voice recordings can be placed on the cine film. In contrast, recording the fluoroscopic image on videotape (*video*fluoroscopy) permits voice recording simultaneously with the fluoroscopic image and requires less radiation exposure (O'Connor & Ardran, 1976). However, videofluoroscopy is more difficult to frame than cinefluoroscopy. Framing is possible, nonetheless, utilizing a Thalner Electronics Video Counter Timer, which places a number in the corner of the videoscreen, each number reflecting one frame of the videotape. Since video is framed at 30 frames per second, when numbers are placed at the rate of 30 per second, each number represents one frame of the video. Several video cassette recorder players are capable of frame-by-frame or stop motion tape advance. Thus, when a tape with numbered frames is played on one of these recorders, frame-by-frame analysis of the movement pattern is possible, similar to analysis of motion picture film. An additional advantage to *video*fluoroscopy in the analysis of deglutition is the ease of patching any video recorder player into fluoroscopic equipment. Such a hookup need not be permanent, and, in fact, video equipment from the education department of a hospital may be borrowed for the time required (30 to 60 minutes) to complete two to three videofluoroscopic studies. Such equipment is generally available in all hospitals and fluoroscopic units are among the most common types of radiographic equipment. Thus, even many smaller hospitals have the capability to do detailed videofluoroscopic studies of deglutition.

The fluoroscopic procedure designed to examine the details of oral, pharyngeal, and cervical esophageal physiology during swallowing is a modified barium swallow procedure. This is sometimes called a "cookie swallow" test because of the kinds of materials given to the patient. The methodology differs from the traditional upper GI, or barium swallow, in several ways: focus of the study and amount and type of material used in the study.

Focus of the Study

The modified barium swallow assesses oral and pharyngeal transit times during deglutition and pinpoints the motility problems in the oral cavity and pharynx which may cause these times to be slow. The functioning of the cricopharyngeal or pharyngoesophageal juncture is examined, and cervical esophageal peristalsis is evaluated. In contrast, the barium swallow gives information on structural competence in the pharynx and esophagus, particularly the lower two-thirds of the esophagus, with little attention paid to details of physiology in the oral cavity and pharynx. The modified barium swallow is designed to assess not only *whether* the patient is aspirating, but also the *reason* for the aspiration, so appropriate treatment can be initiated. Aspiration may occur for a number of reasons, as defined in Chapter 3, including reduced tongue function, delayed or absent swallowing reflex, reduced laryngeal closure/airway protection, and cricopharyngeal hypertonicity. Each of these etiologies requires a different treatment. One of the major purposes of the modified barium swallow is to define the etiology of any aspiration.

Types and Amounts of Materials Used

Three consistencies of material are used in the modified barium swallow to investigate patient complaints of variable swallowing ability: liquid barium, barium paste (Esophatrast), and material requiring mastication (a cookie coated with Esophatrast). Two swallows of each material are given in the following amounts: ⅓ teaspoon liquid, ⅓ teaspoon paste, and ¼ small cookie coated thinly with barium paste. Weathers, Becker, & Genieser, 1974, describe a special device to present the barium liquid to infants. It is a plastic tube with an end for attachment of an ordinary bottle nipple. A 50cc syringe or a plastic bag with a 450cc volume capacity is attached to the open end. The infant can then suck the liquid without the radiologist's hand entering the field of exposure. Patients with suspected aspiration are given even less material, beginning with liquid, to define the reason for the aspiration while using as little material as possible. Of more than 2,000 studies completed at Northwestern University, no patient has acquired aspiration pneumonia as a result of the procedure. Once the reason for the aspiration is defined, the study is terminated to reduce the amount of material entering the airway. If, however, it is thought that a patient can swallow other consistencies without aspiration, small amounts of these materials are also given.

The importance of giving the patient only *very* small amounts of material cannot be overstressed. In many cases, the patients referred for the videofluoroscopic study are ill, have poor respiratory status, and are aspirating. If any large amount (more than a teaspoon) of barium enters their airway, many complications can result. Only a very small amount of material is needed to make an accurate diagnosis (Rossato & Wrightson, 1977; Schultz et al., 1979).

This differs significantly from the traditional barium swallow which is designed to diagnose lesions and anatomic deformities. During the barium swallow, the goal is to fill the pharynx with material and thus outline the the structures (Bachman, 1963; Haubrich, 1977). Unfortunately, if this technique were used with dysphagic patients, they would aspirate a larger amount of material.

FIGURE 4-1
Patient seated on the platform attached to the fluoroscopy table so that the upper aerodigestive tract can be viewed laterally, as shown in the inset in the lower right hand corner.

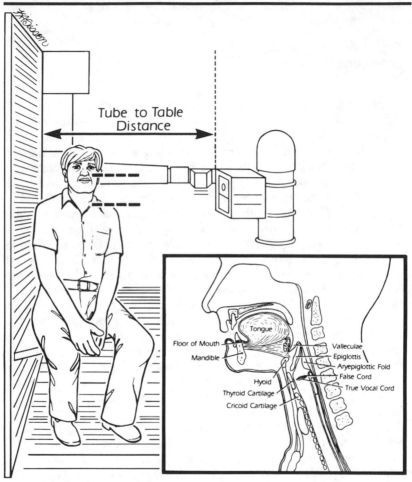

Modified Barium Swallow ("Cookie Swallow") Procedure

Positioning the Patient

Often the most difficult and time-consuming part of the radiographic procedure is positioning the patient. Optimally, the patient should be

FIGURE 4-2
Patient lying on a cart with the head elevated so that the
upper aerodigestive tract can be viewed laterally.

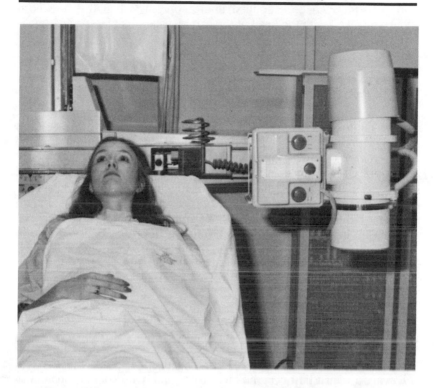

seated and initially viewed in the lateral plane. A patient who is mobile and able to sit without a back rest can be seated on the horizontal platform attached to the fluoroscopy table as shown in Figure 4-1, and raised or lowered to the desired height. Most fluoroscopy machines are fitted with handles so the patient can grip to stabilize his or her position. Initially, then, the patient is seated so that his or her side rests against the table of the fluoroscopy machine and the vocal tract is viewed laterally (Kirchner, 1967; Rossato & Wrightson, 1977).

Some fluoroscopy machines will not accommodate a patient unable to sit unassisted, who needs to sit in a wheelchair or lie on a cart. Because of the design of many types of fluoroscopy equipment, the distance between the tube and the table is not wide enough to fit a wheelchair or cart, as shown in Figure 4-1. Also, many fluoroscopy machines have limited vertical tube movement and can be lowered only a limited distance, usually not low enough to view the patient's laryngopharynx if he or she is seated in a wheelchair. If the fluoroscopy machine accommodates a cart as shown in Figure 4-2, even patients who are unable to walk or sit up independently can be examined fluoroscopically when they are positioned on a cart with the head of the cart elevated to at least a 45° angle.

Focus of the
Fluoroscopic Image

The fluoroscopy tube should focus on the lips anteriorly, the hard palate superiorly, the posterior pharyngeal wall posteriorly, and the bifurcation of the airway and the esophagus inferiorly. Many fluoroscopy machines will permit image magnification. If a patient is suspected of aspirating, it is sometimes helpful to magnify the area around the bifurcation of the airway and the esophagus to get a clear picture of the amount of the aspiration on the first swallow or two. Then the image can be reduced to include the entire vocal tract on the remaining swallows to identify the reason for the aspiration, if it has not already been defined.

Measures and Observations
To Be Made

The lateral view permits a number of measures and observations critical to the identification of the swallowing disorder. First, the oral and pharyngeal transit times can be measured. Oral transit time is defined as the time taken for the movement of the bolus through the oral cavity from the initiation of posterior movement of the bolus by the tongue until the bolus passes the anterior faucial arch. During frame-by-frame measurement of the videotape, a line can be drawn vertically from the base of the tongue upward and can be used as a termination point for the oral phase of the swallow. The pharyngeal phase of the swallow begins when the swallowing reflex triggers and terminates when the bolus passes through the cricopharyngeal juncture. Pharyngeal transit time is defined as the time elasped as the bolus moves between these two points. For measurement from the frame-by-frame videotape, a vertical line drawn from the base of the tongue can be defined as the initial point of pharyngeal transit and a horizontal line drawn through the base of the cricoid cartilage can define the inferior limit of the pharynx or the termination of the pharyngeal transit time.

Esophageal transit time can also be measured but is not usually included in this study because therapeutic intervention for swallowing disorders is not effective in remediating esophageal disorders.

In addition to definition of oral and pharyngeal transit times, the lateral view permits identification of the location of stasis of the bolus along the vocal tract from anterior to posterior. It permits analysis of patterns of lingual movement, gross estimate of the time elapsed before the swallowing reflex triggers, estimate of the amount of vallecular residue after the swallow, and the amount of material aspirated per bolus, as well as the reason for the aspiration. The timing of aspiration relative to the triggering of the swallowing reflex, i.e. before, during, or after the swallow, is also best examined in the lateral view.

When the desired number of swallows of various materials has been completed in the lateral view, the patient can be turned and viewed in the anterior/posterior plane as shown in Figure 4-3 (Ardran & Kemp, 1951). In the A-P view, as the bolus of food or liquid enters the pharynx, it fills the valleculae, giving a scalloped appearance. Then the bolus divides and spills over the aryepiglottic folds into the pyriform sinuses. Usually, the bolus divides fairly equally between the two sides, coming together at about the level of the opening into the esophagus (Ardran & Kemp, 1951). The anterior/posterior view is helpful in looking at asymmetries in function, particularly of the vocal folds, and in viewing residues such as collection of material in the valleculae and residue in the pyriform sinuses. It is more difficult to measure transit times and to observe aspiration in the anterior/posterior view than in the lateral view. In the anterior/posterior view, it is usually best to repeat only swallows of particular materials that exhibit the most severe disturbance in swallowing. This assures that the patient receives a minimal amount of radiation exposure, eliminating repetition of materials which elicit more normal swallows. In the A-P view, it is important to examine the residue in the pharynx after the swallow, comparing the two sides. In the A-P view it is also helpful to tilt the patient's head backwards and ask him to vocalize a continuous *ah* and a rapidly repetitive /a/a/a/ to provide a clear picture of vocal fold movement. Although details of vocal fold movement cannot be examined in this manner, a gross judgment about relative movement of the two cords on adduction and abduction can be made (Bachman, 1963; Maguire, 1966). This is often helpful to the clinician in assessing the patient's ability to close his or her vocal folds and protect the airway during the swallow.

Instructions to the Patient

When the patient is positioned, it should be explained that he or she will be asked to swallow three different materials: two liquid swallows, two

FIGURE 4-3
Patient seated on the platform attached to the fluoroscopy table so that the upper aerodigestive tract can be viewed anterior-posteriorly, as shown in the inset in the lower right hand corner.

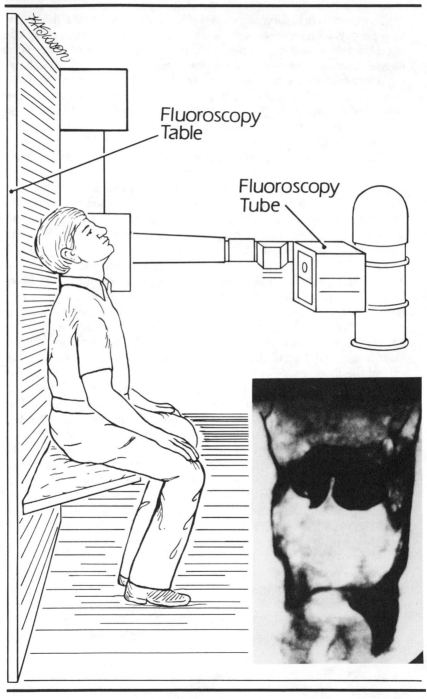

paste or pudding swallows, and two swallows of a small piece of cookie with barium on top. It is explained that only very small amounts of each material will be given on any swallow, and that if he or she has difficulty he or she should cough and/or spit out the material if necessary. However, it should be emphasized that the patient should try his or her best throughout the examination.

Materials To Be Swallowed

The liquid barium is generally the first material used and is presented on a teaspoon. Approximately ⅓ of a teaspoon is used for each swallow. The patient is asked to hold the material in his or her mouth until the examiner is ready and then told to swallow the material when ready. Liquid is the first material presented even if the patient is known to aspirate, because it is usually best to define the reason for aspiration and the amount of aspiration during the first several swallows. Liquids are often most easily aspirated and yet are least apt to block the airway creating increased fear in the patient.

If the patient aspirates a large amount of each liquid swallow, the examiner may decide not to proceed with the rest of the swallows. This decision is usually based on the reason for the aspiration. For example, if it is determined that poor tongue control or a delayed swallowing reflex is the reason for the aspiration, it may be that material of a slightly thicker consistency will not be aspirated as easily, so swallows of the thicker material can be attempted. If successful, the patient can then be placed on a diet of that consistency while therapy is directed toward improving the physiology for liquid swallows. If, on the other hand, the patient's aspiration is a result of reduced laryngeal closure *during* the swallow so material falls directly through the larynx and into the airway *during* the swallow, it is unlikely a different texture of material will affect this aspiration, and the examiner may decide to terminate the study after liquids, withholding all oral feeding while therapy is directed toward improving laryngeal closure. If the aspiration occurs *after* the swallow because of residue in the valleculae or pyriform sinuses, the patient may not do as well on swallows of thicker material. Greater peristalsis is generally necessary to clear thicker materials from the pharynx and the cricopharyngeal opening must be greater for pastes than liquid materials, as liquids can slowly drain through a slightly opened P-E segment. If these problems are present the examiner may decide to terminate the study after liquid swallows, knowing that the patient will do less well on swallows of thicker material.

After the liquid swallows, two swallows of barium in a pudding consistency are usually given. Again, the amount is ⅓ of a teaspoon, The material used is Esophatrast which comes in a large, toothpaste-like tube.

If the patient is unable to take liquid or paste material from a spoon, a syringe may be used to place liquid into the posterior oral cavity and a tongue blade can be used to wipe material of a thicker consistency onto the back of the tongue.

The third material used is ¼ of a butter cookie or a Lorna Doone with a light coating of the Esophatrast paste as a contrast medium. On these last two swallows, the patient is asked to chew the material well and to initiate the swallow when he or she is ready. The directions are slightly different from the previous swallows in which the patient was asked to wait for the investigator's command to begin the swallow. In the case of the masticated material, the patient is told to go ahead and swallow as soon as he or she has completed chewing.

Trial Therapy

When the swallowing study is completed, the physiologic details of deglutition should have been clearly delineated. The clinician can then decide on the nature of treatment for the specific swallowing disorder. If the proposed therapy technique is a relatively simple one, for example postural changes, the examiner may wish to attempt trial therapy in the presence of videofluoroscopy (O'Connor & Ardran, 1976). In this case, the clinician can ask the patient to position his or her head in a particular way or to follow specific instructions while swallowing and examine the results on videofluoroscopy, comparing the physiology to the earlier examination results. Often, postural changes may result in dramatic changes in physiology, as described in Chapter 5, and may permit the patient to begin oral intake. Therefore, it is very helpful when these changes are documented on fluoroscopy. In general, a maximum of three additional swallows are completed while attempting therapeutic techniques so the total number of swallows during fluoroscopy is 6 to 10. The exposure time is generally less than 5 minutes and presents less radiation exposure to the patient than would be received during a standard radiographic procedure such as a barium swallow or lower GI series.

Guidelines for
Videofluoroscopy Referral

In general, any patient who is aspirating, whose swallowing disorder is of pharyngeal origin, or who has a pharyngeal component should be referred for a videofluoroscopic study. As discussed later in this chapter, the bedside clinical examination can define swallowing disorders arising in the oral cavity, but can only *infer* pharyngeal disorders. In addition, many patients who aspirate will not be identified at bedside because they give no sign of the aspiration. In a recent study, the results of the bedside examination of swallowing were compared with the data from video-fluoroscopic examinations of deglutition on the same patients who aspirated. Approximately 40% of the patients who aspirated regularly during the videofluoroscopic study were not identified as aspirating when examined at the bedside, because they did not cough or give any other outward sign of aspiration. This is particularly true of neurologic patients, whose sensitivity may be reduced.

Who Should Do the Videofluoroscopic Study

Typically, it is best if the swallowing therapist and the radiologist collaborate in performing the study. Each brings particular expertise to the analyses of the swallowing disorder. The radiologist is trained to identify structural abnormalities, but, typically, has minimal knowledge of the details of oral and pharyngeal movement patterns during deglutition. The swallowing therapist is familiar with these movement patterns and the therapeutic regimens to treat particular disorders. The combination of skills of the two professionals results in optimum diagnosis and management decisions.

Videofluoroscopic Study Report

The report of the study should be written and signed by all professionals involved. Typically, it begins with a description of the patient's symptoms or complaints. Then, measures of oral transit time should be given for each material swallowed, followed by a description of any neuro-muscular or anatomic problems observed in the oral phase of the swallow. Any variability in deglutition with the three consistencies of material should be noted.

Pharyngeal transit times should then be specified, noting variations with consistency of material. Any anatomic or neuromuscular problems observed in the pharyngeal phase of the swallow should be described. Amount of aspiration on particular food consistencies, and the etiology of the aspiration should be noted. Amount of vallecular residue should also be defined. Finally, recommendations should be outlined regarding: (a) management of oral feeding and (b) procedures for swallowing therapy. These should include recommendations for consultations by other professionals.

The Bedside Clinical Examination

The bedside clinical examination is designed to provide the clinician with the following data for use in diagnosis and treatment planning: (a) information on the history of the patient's disorder including the person's awareness of his or her swallowing disorder and indications of the localization and nature of the disorder; (b) the patient's medical status including nutritional and respiratory status, i.e. presence of a nasogastric feeding tube or gastrostomy and placement of a cuffed or uncuffed tracheostomy tube; (c) the patient's oral anatomy; (d) the patient's labial control as this may affect keeping food in his or her mouth; (e) the patient's lingual control as it may affect oral manipulation of food and the posterior transit of food through the oral cavity; (f) the patient's palatal function as it may affect entrance of food into his or her nose during the swallow; (g) the patient's pharyngeal control as it may affect movement of food through the pharynx or may cause aspiration after the swallow; (h) the patient's laryngeal control as it may affect airway protection and aspiration during the swallow; (i) the patient's general ability to follow directions; (j) the best combination of instructions that will facilitate the patient's normal swallow; and (k) the patient's symptoms during attempts to swallow (Griffin, 1974; Linden & Siebins, 1980). The clinical examination can be divided into two parts: (1) the preparatory examination, with no actual swallows, and (2) the initial swallowing examination when actual swallowing is attempted and physiology is observed.

Preparatory Examination

The preparatory examination begins with collection of information from the patient's chart and includes a complete examination of vocal tract control (Griffin, 1974).

Patient Chart
Examination

Initially, the swallowing therapist should carefully examine the patient's medical chart to determine the individual's respiratory status, including any reports or comments on pulmonary function testing and/or the presence of a tracheostomy tube (cuffed or uncuffed). Also, information on the history of the patient's swallowing problem, including duration, the patient's general medical status, ability to follow directions, motivation, and other aspects of the patient's general behavior are helpful to the therapist prior to beginning the bedside examination. The nutritional status (oral feeding versus nasogastric tube or gastrostomy) should also be determined from the patient's medical chart.

Observations upon Entering
the Patient's Room

As the clinician enters the patient's room, several observations should be made automatically: The patient's posture in bed, his or her alertness and reaction to the clinician's entrance, the presence or absence of a tracheostomy tube and its status (cuff inflated or deflated), and the patient's general handling of his or her own secretions and management of the tube itself. During the initial part of the bedside examination as the history is being taken, the clinician should be making informal observations on the patient's ability to follow directions and answer questions, as well as the individual's general alertness. Throughout this time, the clinician should also be observing the patient's management of secretions and of the tracheostomy tube, if present.

Tracheostomy Tubes. Tracheostomy tubes are normally placed for: (1) upper airway obstruction above the level of the true vocal folds; or (2) potential upper airway obstruction such as may be created by edema following oral, pharyngeal, or laryngeal surgery. The tube is generally inserted into the trachea through a surgical incision made between the third and fourth tracheal rings. This placement well below the true vocal cords avoids damage to the larynx. Occasionally in emergency situations tracheostomas are placed higher than the second tracheal ring and may cause laryngeal scarring after removal. Tubes are usually left in place until the airway obstruction or the potential for airway obstruction is passed. Occasionally tracheostomy tubes remain permanently.

FIGURE 4-4
The parts of a tracheostomy tube.

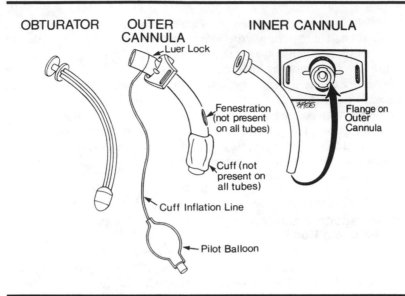

Tracheostomy tubes generally have three parts as illustrated in Figure 4-4: an outer cannula, an inner cannula, and an obturator. In normal use, the outer cannula always stays in place, the inner cannula remains in the tube except for cleaning, and the obturator is inserted only to provide a smooth, rounded tip for the initial insertion of the tracheostomy tube. The outer cannula remains in place to hold the tracheostomy site open until it can be allowed to close. When patients are being weaned from tracheostomy tubes, two procedures are used. First, the tube (most often a size 8) will be changed to a smaller size to encourage oral/nasal breathing in combination with breathing through the tracheostomy site. If the smaller tube (often a size 4) is tolerated well it will be plugged with a cork for periods of time to assess the patient's ability to maintain oral/nasal breathing without distress before the tube is removed altogether.

Normally, there is a small amount of space between the tracheostomy tube and the walls of the trachea, as seen in Figure 4-5a. When the patient inhales and occludes the outer end of the tracheostomy tube with a finger, air can pass around the tube and through the larynx, and produce voice (Figure 4-5b). Because the amount of air passing between the tube and the walls of the trachea is reduced from normal, voice will often be softer and more breathy in quality than normal.

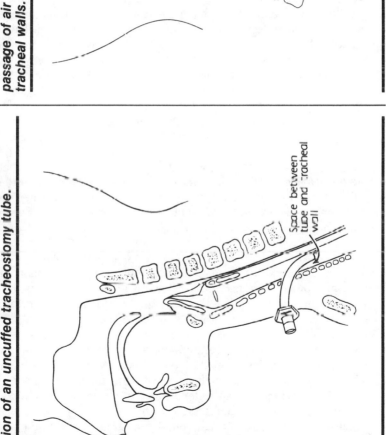

FIGURE 4-5a
Mid-sagittal section of the head and neck showing the position of an uncuffed tracheostomy tube.

Space between tube and tracheal wall

FIGURE 4-5b
Mid-sagittal section of the head and neck showing the passage of air between the tracheostomy tube and the tracheal walls.

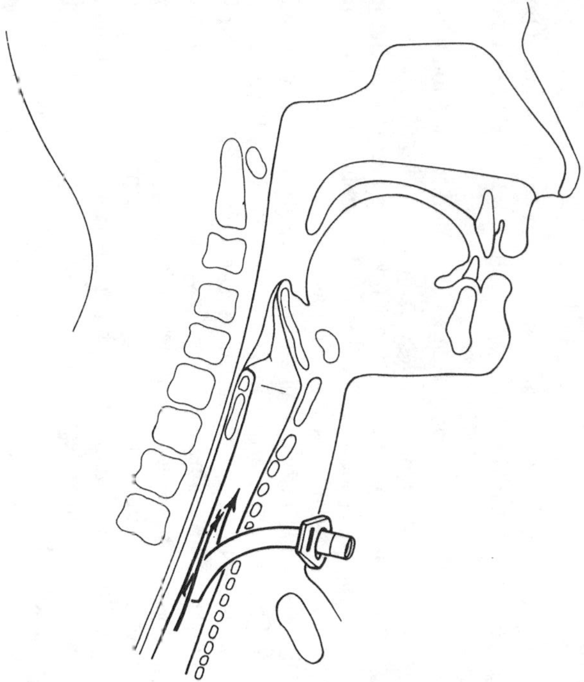

There are two important variations in tracheostomy tubes. A tracheostomy tube may be cuffed or uncuffed, fenestrated or unfenestrated.

Cuffed tracheostomy tubes. A cuffed tracheostomy tube (shown in Figure 4-6) is sometimes placed when there is potential for the patient to aspirate material. The cuff surrounds the inner end of the tracheostomy tube like a balloon. When the cuff is deflated as in Figure 4-6, the tracheostomy tube is the same as if it had no cuff, i.e. there is space between the tracheal wall and the tube so that air may pass upward as indicated by the arrow in Figure 4-7. When inflated as in Figure 4-8, however, the cuff contacts the tracheal wall, preventing air from passing upward and sealing the lower airway from secretions from above. Thus, with the cuff inflated, no material from above the larynx can pass through into the trachea and bronchi. The cuff is inflated for patients who are aspirating to prevent aspiration pneumonia. Saliva, food, and other secretions will then collect above the cuff. When the cuff is deflated in this situation, therefore, thorough suctioning is necessary to catch material draining around the tube into the airway. Cuffed tracheostomy tubes are generally not left in place for a long time, as the pressure of the cuff contacting the tracheal wall can create tracheal irritation. This can occur even though cuffs are designed to create minimal pressure against the tracheal wall. Also, an inflated tracheostomy cuff may inhibit a patient's relearning to swallow by restricting laryngeal elevation (Bonanno, 1971), reducing laryngeal sensitivity (Feldman, Deal, & Urquhart, 1966) or placing pressure on the esophagus via the common posterior wall between the trachea and the esophagus. It should also be noted that occasionally a cuffed tracheostomy tube will not completely occlude the trachea because of tracheal wall deviations or misfit tubes resulting in some aspiration past the cuffed tube.

Fenestrated tracheostomy tubes. If a patient is having difficulty producing voice with a normal tracheostomy tube, a fenestration, or window, may be cut into the tube to allow for greater air flow, as shown in Figures 4-9 and 4-10. Often this fenestration is made only in the outer cannula so when the patient wants to talk he or she removes the inner cannula. When the inner cannula is placed into the tracheostomy tube, the fenestration is closed. Fenestrated tubes may be used with patients who are close to being weaned from the tracheostomy tube or in patients whose communication is ineffective with the small amount of airflow generally possible with an unfenestrated tube. It is rare for a cuffed tracheostomy tube to be fenestrated, as the fenestration would negate the occlusive effects of the inflated cuff. A fenestration might be made in a cuffed tube, however, if a patient no longer needs the cuff inflated.

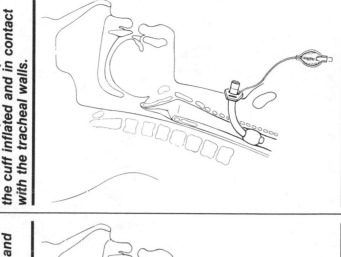

FIGURE 4-8
Mid-sagittal section of the head and neck showing the cuffed tracheostomy tube in place with the cuff inflated and in contact with the tracheal walls.

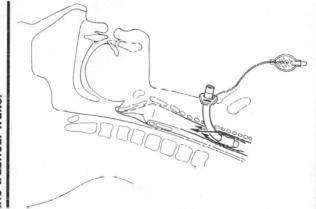

FIGURE 4-7
Mid-sagittal section of the head and neck showing the passage of air between the tracheostomy tube with the cuff deflated and the tracheal walls.

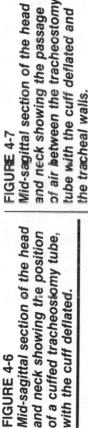

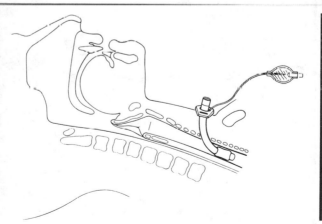

FIGURE 4-6
Mid-sagittal section of the head and neck showing the position of a cuffed tracheostomy tube, with the cuff deflated.

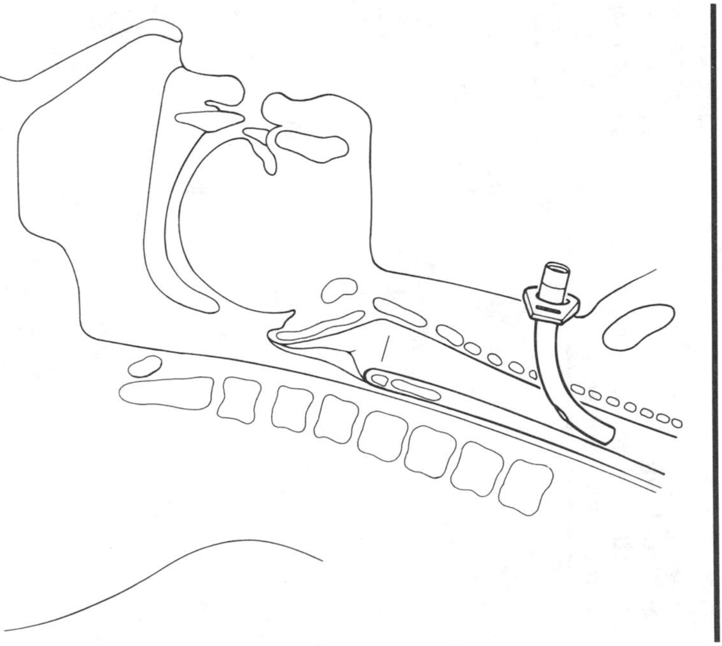

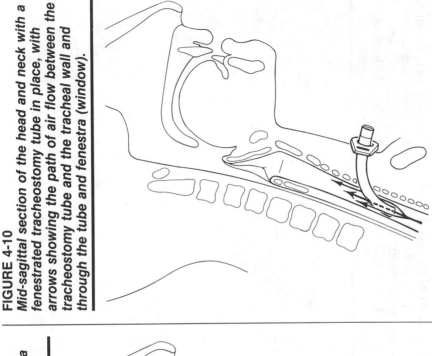

FIGURE 4-10
Mid-sagittal section of the head and neck with a fenestrated tracheostomy tube in place, with arrows showing the path of air flow between the tracheostomy tube and the tracheal wall and through the tube and fenestra (window).

FIGURE 4-9
Mid-sagittal section of the head and neck with a fenestrated tracheostomy tube in place.

History

It is important to gather information from the patient if possible, or family or nursing staff if the patient is unable to give a sufficient report, regarding the exact nature of the patient's swallowing disorder (Dobie, 1978; Donald & Dawes, 1977; Edwards, 1970; Griffin & Tollison, 1980; Griffin, 1974; Kirchner, 1967; McConchie, 1973; O'Connor & Ardran, 1976; Phillips & Hendrix, 1971; Pitcher, 1973). When did the disorder begin? Did it worsen gradually or rapidly? How does the problem vary with different consistencies of food, i.e. liquid, pudding, and solid food, particularly meat? What specifically happens when the patient tries to swallow? Does material stop somewhere along the way? If so, where? High or low in the throat? Does the patient cough and choke? If food collects, can the patient point to the spot in his or her mouth or throat where he or she feels material collect?

Studies have shown patients who are aware a disorder is present to be highly reliable in their identification and description of a swallowing disorder. However, if a patient denies having a swallowing disorder, the individual is frequently in error and often has a problem, sometimes severe in nature, to which he or she is oblivious. Typically, if a patient points to the base of the tongue area or the epiglottis and indicates that material has collected at that point, or the individual feels material "stuck" in his or her throat at that point, the material is likely to be hesitating in the valleculae at the base of the tongue. If, however, the patient points lower on the neck, just below the larynx, and indicates material is sticking there, material is usually collecting in the pyriform sinuses because of a dysfunctioning cricopharyngeus muscle. Coughing and choking, when present, generally indicate aspiration or entry of material into the patient's airway.

The pattern of difficulty with particular consistencies of food is also helpful information for the clinician. Because in therapy it is generally best to start with easiest consistencies, it's important to know which consistency the patient feels is easiest to swallow. Particular swallowing disorders present differing symptoms as related to consistency of material. For example, patients with difficulty in oral transit because of poor control of the tongue may find liquids easiest to swallow, but pastes and thicker materials very difficult. Conversely, patients who have very delayed or absent triggering of the swallowing reflex will generally do best with materials of a thicker consistency that tend to cling to the pharynx and the valleculae until the reflex triggers, and will have greater difficulty with liquids because these splash into the pharynx and the airway before the reflex has triggered. There are no hard and fast rules, however, which tell the clinician that a particular disorder always presents with a particular pattern of difficulty with particular food consistencies. This is especially true for patients with multiple swallowing disorders that affect both the oral and pharyngeal stages of the swallow.

In many cases, when the patient describes his or her problem with swallowing, it is important to ask the patient to demonstrate what he or she did when starting to swallow. In these demonstrations it often becomes clear that the patient took too much material, positioned it inappropriately in the mouth, or utilized an instrument or utensil which he or she could not manage well. The patient does not actually need to swallow the food or liquid. Simply repeating the motions leading to the swallow will give the clinician much information.

On the basis of a careful history, the swallowing therapist may have information on: (1) the localization of the disorder in terms of the oral or pharyngeal stage of the swallow, or both; (2) the kind of material easiest for the patient to swallow and the most difficult type; and (3) some indication of the nature of the swallowing disorder.

The Examination
of Oral Anatomy

This examination should include careful observation of lip configuration, palatal configuration (height and width), soft palate and uvular dimensions relative to the distance to the posterior pharyngeal wall, intact nature of the faucial arches (both anterior and posterior), lingual configuration, and the adequacy of the sulci at the sides and front of the mandible. Any scarring in the oral cavity or on the neck and any asymmetries in structures should be very carefully examined. When the anatomical examination has been completed, the functional assessment should begin.

Oral Motor Control
Examination

The oral-motor examination should include evaluation of the range, rate, and accuracy of movement of the lips, tongue, and soft palate during speech, reflexive activity, and swallowing (Dobie, 1978).

Labial Function. The examination of labial function should include the following tasks: spreading the lips as widely as possible on the vowel /i/, rounding them as much as possible on the vowel /u/, rapidly alternating these two postures (/i/ and /u/) approximately 10 times, rapidly repeating the syllable *pa* to determine a diadochokinetic rate, closing the mouth tightly and observing the patient's labial closure during rest and during saliva swallowing. The patient should also be asked to repeat a sentence that includes a large number of bilabial stop phonemes, with the completeness of bilabial closure to be examined on each articulation.

For chewing, the clinician should be concerned about the patient's ability to maintain lip closure despite changes in head posture and movements of the jaw in manipulating food. The clinician may ask the patient to move his or her jaw and maintain lip closure, or may ask the patient to shape his or her lips around a straw, spoon, or fork.

Lingual Function. Lingual function should be assessed both anteriorly and posteriorly. For *anterior tongue examination,* the patient should be asked to: (1) extend the tongue tip as far forward as possible and retract it as far backward as possible; (2) touch each corner of his or her mouth and then rapidly alternate the lateral movements; (3) open the mouth widely and with the mouth in this position elevate the tongue tip to the alveolar ridge, and rapidly alternate elevation and depression of the tongue tip while maintaining an open mouth; (4) rapidly repeat the syllable /ta/ to determine a diadochokinetic rate; (5) repeat a sentence containing a number of tip-alveolar stop consonants and assess the completeness of tongue tip to alveolar ridge contact during these productions, including lateral seal on the lateral alveolus; and (6) reach the sulci between cheeks and lower alveolus and reach the anterior sulci between lip and anterior alveolus. The patient should also be asked to slide his or her tongue along the palatal vault from the very front near the alveolar ridge toward the back, as if clearing food from the palate. The patient may also be asked to manipulate one end of a piece of licorice whip with his or her tongue while the other end is held by the clinician.

Posterior tongue function can be assessed by asking the patient to: (1) lift the back of the tongue as if saying a /k/ and holding the back of the tongue elevated in this position for several seconds; (2) repeat the syllable /ka/ as rapidly as possible to assess a diadochokinetic rate; (3) repeat a sentence containing a number of back velar stop phonemes to determine the completeness of tongue-to-palate contact during these productions.

Soft Palate Function and Oral Reflexes. Function of the soft palate can be examined by asking the patient to produce a strong, loud /a/ and to sustain that sound for several seconds (Dobie, 1978). The patient may also rapidly repeat the /a/. The clinician should note the action of the levator muscle in elevation of the palate and the palato-pharyngeus muscle in retraction of the palate. The palatal and gag reflexes should also be tested. To elicit the palatal reflex, a cold instrument, such as the head of a size 00 laryngeal mirror (¼″ diameter) may be contacted against the juncture of the hard and soft palates or the inferior edge of the soft palate and uvula (DeJong, 1967), as shown in Figure 4-11. This contact should elicit an upward and backward movement of the soft palate, but no reaction in the pharyngeal walls. The palatal reflex stimulates soft palate movement but does not generate the total pharyngeal response of a gag reflex. In a recent study of oral reflexes (Jenkins, Lazarus, & Logemann, 1982), the palatal reflex was found to be the least stable of the oral reflexes, often requiring two strokes to elicit it. Neurologically, the afferent portion of the reflex seems to be carried through the glossopharyngeal (and possibly, the vagus nerve) while the efferent portion of the reflex seems to be carried through the vagus nerve (and possibly the glossopharyngeal). The trigeminal nerve, which also innervates part of the palate, may be involved in this reflex.

The gag reflex should be elicited by contacting the head of a laryngeal mirror against the base of the tongue or the posterior pharyngeal wall. A strong contraction of the entire pharyngeal wall and soft palate should be observed as a result of this contact. While many individuals with normal swallowing ability demonstrate reduced or absent gag reflexes (DeJong, 1967), many health care professionals erroneously consider the presence or absence of a gag reflex in neurologically impaired patients as an indication of the patient's ability to swallow. There are no data to support this relationship. The afferent impulses for the gag reflex are carried mainly by X, although IX may be involved (DeJong, 1967).

Oral Sensitivity Examination. The oral sensitivity examination should include an assessment of light touch. The clinician needs to identify any areas in the mouth that have reduced sensitivity. There are no clear guidelines for interpretation of oral sensitivity testing, thus, the clinician can only compare the various areas of the patient's oral cavity to identify locations with greatest sensitivity and those least sensitive. With a cotton swab, the clinician can make light contact at various points along the tongue, from anterior to posterior, along the buccal mucosa, and at the base and up the faucial arches, to determine the patient's awareness of light touch. This information will have impact on the clinician's placement of food in the oral cavity, as all food should be positioned at the point of maximum sensitivity.

Management Information To Be Collected from the Oral Examination. The results of the labial assessment should alert the clinician to any facial paralysis and any problem the patient may have in maintaining

FIGURE 4-11
Frontal and lateral views of the oral cavity and pharynx, with areas sensitive to triggering of the palatal, gag and swallowing reflexes identified.

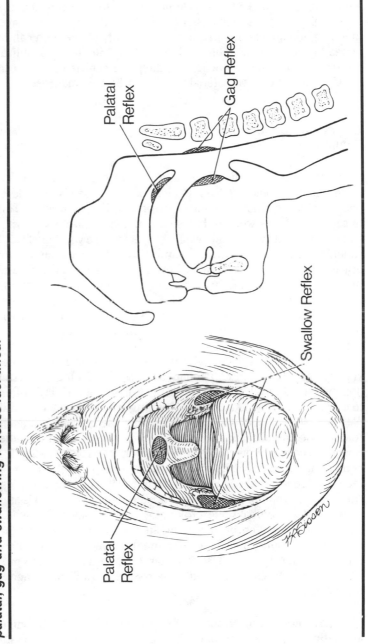

Logemann

lip closure when food is placed in the mouth. The lingual function examination should identify any limitation in tongue function that may affect ability to propel food posteriorly or to hold food in a cohesive bolus; therefore, identifying the area in the oral cavity where food can be positioned for best tongue control (Griffin, 1974). Similarly, identification of impairments in tongue function will help the clinician to select the particular consistencies of material which can be best managed.

Laryngeal Function Examination

Examination of *laryngeal function* should begin with assessment of voice quality (Dobie, 1978). A patient with hoarseness should be suspected of having reduced laryngeal closure during the swallow. This is not to say that patients who are hoarse automatically have swallowing problems, but patients with swallowing disorders whose vocal quality is hoarse should have a careful laryngeal examination. Referral to an otolaryngologist for indirect laryngoscopy is warranted. In addition, the swallowing therapist should examine laryngeal diadochokinetic rates i.e. rapid repetition of the syllable /ha/, listening for clear production of the vowel and voiceless production of the *h*. Some types of neurologically impaired patients will tend to produce a single intermediate adduction of the larynx with a continuous breathy /ha/ as the result instead of individual *ha* syllables. The patient should also be asked to cough as hard as possible and to clear the throat as strongly as possible. During these tasks, the therapist should evaluate the apparent strength and quality of the cough to determine its potential for expectorating aspirated material. Asking the patient to slide up and down scale evaluates the function of the cricothyroid muscle and intrinsic muscles of the vocal cords, and tests the superior laryngeal nerve as it innervates the cricothyroid muscle. Since the swallowing reflex may trigger from the superior laryngeal nerve, as may the cough reflex, inability to change pitch may imply reduced sensitivity within and surrounding the larynx. Phonation time tasks, that is asking the patient to take a breath and prolong a *z* for as long as possible on the subsequent exhalation or to prolong an *s* on the subsequent exhalation, can provide some information on the relative control of the larynx. Phonation time is also a test of respiration, so during these prolonged articulations, the clinician should observe chest wall movement during the exhalation.

Management Information To Be Collected from the Laryngeal Examination: On the basis of the laryngeal control examination, the clinician should have some suspicion about the involvement of laryngeal function in the swallowing disorder. If laryngeal function appears to be borderline, the clinician may decide to teach the patient the supraglottic swallow in an attempt to increase the patient's airway protection prior to initiating any swallows. This technique is discussed in Chapter 5.

Pulmonary Function Testing

Pulmonary function testing helps the clinician determine whether the patient can tolerate any amount of aspiration. This test battery is ordered and interpreted by a physician. The information provided should be used when contemplating oral feeding regimens that may involve some degree of aspiration. There are currently no data that indicate how much aspiration a patient may tolerate before contracting aspiration pneumonia. There are also no guidelines on the level of pulmonary function that must be present in order for a patient to tolerate some degree of aspiration. Thus, each physician must establish his or her own guidelines to determine when oral feeding in the presence of aspiration is acceptable. Many physicians have found pulmonary function data helpful in making this determination.

Information Collected from the Preparatory Examination

On the basis of the preparatory portion of the bedside clinical examination, the swallowing therapist should have the following information: (1) the posture that may result in best swallowing, (2) the best position of food in the mouth, (3) the best food consistency, and (4) an indication of the sequence of swallowing instructions that may result in most normal swallowing, in addition to some indication of the nature of the patient's swallowing disorder.

Decisions on Best Posture

Posture can be of great assistance in the management of swallowing disorders. The evaluation may have indicated poor tongue control, with the patient having difficulty maneuvering the bolus in his or her mouth,

FIGURE 4-12
*Mid-sagittal view of the head and neck, with the head
extended backward, illustrating the disappearance of the
vallecular space in this position.*

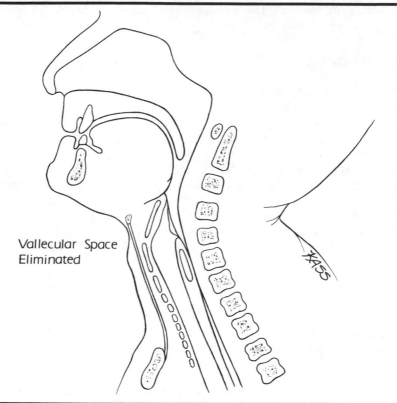

Vallecular Space
Eliminated

or the bolus trickling over the base of the tongue and into the pharynx
before the voluntary swallow is initiated. In such a case, it may be best to
ask the patient to tilt his or her head downward as food is introduced
in the mouth and then throw his or her head backward to drain material
from the mouth when the patient is ready to initiate the swallow, as shown
in Figure 4-12. Tilting the head backward is an entirely safe technique if
the patient has normal pharyngeal and laryngeal control. Under those
circumstances airway protection will be adequate. If, on the basis of the
careful history, the patient is known to have had a hemilaryngectomy, or
any reason for a delay in triggering of the swallowing reflex, it may be

FIGURE 4-13
*Mid-sagittal view of the head and neck, with the head down,
illustrating the enhancement of the vallecular space in this
position.*

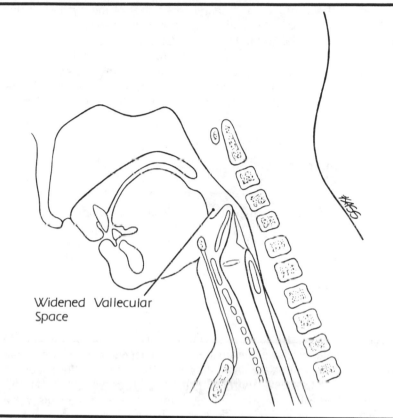

Widened Vallecular
Space

helpful to tilt his or her head downward so that the vallecular space is
widened, as shown in Figure 4-13. With this position, material will rest in
the valleculae long enough to facilitate triggering of the reflex, and the
valleculae will divert material away from the airway. Similarly, if patients
have slightly inadequate laryngeal closure, the forward tilting of the head
may result in greater protection of the airway by the overhanging epiglottis. If, according to the history and medical examination, the patient
exhibits a pharyngeal paralysis, it may be helpful to turn the patient's head
toward the affected side to close the pyriform sinus on that side, directing

material down the more functional side (Kirchner, 1967). If on the other hand, a patient has a lingual hemiparesis or reduction in oral function on one side in addition to involvement of the pharynx on that side, tilting the head toward the stronger side may result in directing the material down that side, in both the oral and pharyngeal stages of the swallow. If that technique is necessary, the patient will generally need to tilt his or her head before food is placed in the mouth. Otherwise, with the head in the normal position material will tend to fall toward the affected side. These postural decisions should be made prior to initiating the first swallow with the patient and should be based on the information collected in the preswallowing evaluation, including careful history-taking and chart review.

Selection of Food Position in the Mouth

Positioning food in the mouth should depend on information on oral sensitivity and oral function. In general, food should be positioned on the side of greater function and greater sensitivity. If liquid must be placed posteriorly in the oral cavity, a straw used as a pipette, or a syringe may be used. A tongue blade is often helpful in positioning thicker foods in particular places on the tongue.

Selection of Best Food Consistency. Selection of food texture to use in the actual swallowing evaluation should depend on: (1) information collected in the history, (2) data on oral control, and (3) information on pharyngeal and laryngeal control. In general, patients with poor oral control will do best with liquid or materials of thin consistency; patients with a delayed swallowing reflex will do best with materials of a thicker consistency, such as applesauce or mashed potatoes; patients with reduced pharyngeal peristalsis will do best with liquids; patients with reduced functioning of the cricopharyngeus muscle will do better with liquids; and patients with reduced laryngeal closure will do best with materials of a thicker consistency. Combinations of disorders, however, make selection of material more difficult. For example, a patient with a disturbance in oral function and delayed swallowing reflex, may do best with a consistency somewhere between liquid and paste. Thus, gravity can assist oral propulsion of the bolus during the oral phase of the swallow, but material will tend to cling to the valleculae and epiglottis while waiting for the reflex to trigger, rather than splashing into the pharynx and the

FIGURE 4-14
A size #00 laryngeal mirror to be used for stimulation of the swallowing reflex.

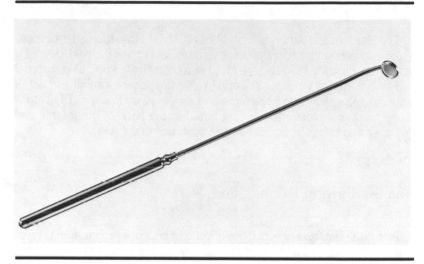

larynx. The swallowing therapist should give careful consideration to selection of consistency of materials prior to initiating any swallows.

Selection of Optimum Swallowing Instructions

When a patient is first asked to swallow, he or she should be given a series of instructions designed to elicit the most normal swallow possible. The sequence of swallowing instructions should be based on information collected in the preparatory examination. Posture or sequence of postures should be carefully noted as should the need for voluntary protection of the airway during the swallow. For example, the patient with slightly reduced tongue control and reduced laryngeal control may need to begin by tilting his or her head downward while putting food in his or her mouth, then tip his or her head backward when he or she is going to swallow, and hold his or her breath during the swallow to voluntarily protect the airway. There may be a total of five or seven steps in a sequence of swallowing instructions. Details of this sequence will vary from patient to patient and are entirely dependent on results of the preparatory clinical examination.

Logemann

Utensils To Be
Used in the Initial
Swallowing Evaluation

The clinician should bring a number of utensils into the patient's room for the swallowing evaluation. These include: (1) a #0 or 00 laryngeal mirror, as illustrated in Figure 4-14, (2) a tongue blade for wiping material onto the posterior tongue, (3) a cup to give the patient a small amount of material, (4) a spoon for presenting liquids and paste material, (5) a straw to be used as a pipette for placing liquid in the back of the mouth, and (6) a syringe to squirt liquid into the posterior oral cavity.

The Swallowing Examination

Prior to initiating any actual swallows, the patient's preparation is most important. If the patient is exhibiting any excess secretions, suctioning should be completed both orally and transtracheostomy, if a tracheostomy tube is present.

Management of the
Tracheostomy Tube

When working with swallowing, it is generally best to *deflate the tracheostomy cuff prior to attempting any swallows.* An inflated cuff may irritate the trachea as the larynx elevates during swallowing. Or, the inflated cuff may restrict laryngeal elevation.

However, before proceeding with swallowing or with deflating the cuff, the clinician should *check with the patient's physician* and obtain his or her assessment of the advisability of deflating the cuff, as well as the patient's tolerance for possible aspiration, even in small amounts.

It is important to remember to *suction the patient well both orally and via the tracheostomy* to assure a clear oral cavity and airway prior to beginning therapy. It is particularly necessary to *suction the patient well immediately after the cuff is deflated* so any secretions sitting above the cuff will be cleared away as they drain around the tube and into the trachea. This suctioning is usually best done by nursing staff, trained in suction techniques rather than the swallowing therapist. However for emergencies, the swallowing therapist should know how to suction orally and transtracheostomy. If the nurse participates in this procedure, he or she will be able to observe the patient's swallowing training and can then reinforce the process with the patient throughout the day.

During each swallow, the patient should *occlude his or her tracheostomy tube* with a finger to establish as near normal tracheal pressure as possible. This step should be incorporated into the sequence of instructions for swallowing.

There are several advantages to initiating swallowing therapy with a tracheostomy tube in place. First, the swallowing therapist can observe aspiration more directly by examining any expectoration through the tube. At the same time, elimination of aspirated material by coughing or suction is accomplished more easily. Several authors report specific but rarely occurring problems related to the presence of tracheostomy tubes during swallowing therapy: (1) restriction of upward laryngeal movement to protect the airway by anchoring the trachea to the strap muscles and skin of the neck along a tract of cicatrix or scar tissue thus increasing the chances of aspiration (Bonanno, 1971; Pinkus, 1973); (2) compression of the esophagus by the tube pushing posteriorly on the common wall between the trachea and the esophagus (particularly true of cuffed tracheostomy tubes) (Betts, 1965; Pinkus, 1973); and (3) the change in intratracheal pressure because of the presence of the tube. Of the over 2,000 patients treated at Northwestern University for swallowing problems, only one patient's swallowing disorder could be attributed to the tracheostomy tube. For the majority of patients in swallowing therapy, the advantages of a tracheostomy outweight the disadvantages. However, swallowing problems related directly to tracheostomy do occur occasionally and should be considered in tracheotomized patients with dysphagia.

Prior to actually asking the patient to swallow, his or her particular set of directions should be reviewed with the patient and written down. The patient should be given an opportunity to practice several dry swallows according to this sequence. In general, patients do best if they are given adequate time to absorb the instructions and review them with the therapist before actually trying to swallow any food or liquid. Coaching by the therapist as the patient proceeds through the sequence is very helpful. Once the patient has demonstrated an ability to follow the outlined instructions, several actual swallows can be tried. It is usually advisable to assure the patient that the amount he or she will be given to swallow will be minimal. The patient should be encouraged to cough whenever necessary but to do the best he or she can throughout the swallowing sequence. It's also helpful to reassure the patient that the small amount of material to be swallowed should prevent difficulty with breathing during or after the swallow. And again, coughing should be reinforced as it clears the airway. Occasionally, patients feel that coughing indicates poor performance and try to consciously inhibit coughing to show how well they are doing.

Approximately the same amounts of material as used in radiographic studies should be used for the bedside examination. That is, ⅓ of a teaspoon of liquid, ⅓ of a teaspoon of the paste or pudding-like consistency, and ½ of a cookie, if masticated material is to be used. These small amounts of material are not sufficient to block a patient's airway and, if aspirated, should cause minimal difficulty.

Observations during the Trial Swallows

During the swallow, it is helpful for the clinician to place his or her hand under the patient's chin with fingers spread, as illustrated in Figure 4-15. The index finger should be positioned immediately behind the mandible anteriorly, the middle finger at the hyoid bone, the third finger at the top of the thyroid cartilage, and the fourth finger at the bottom of the thyroid cartilage. In this way, submandibular movement, hyoid movement, and laryngeal movement can be assessed during the swallow. No pressure should be placed on the tissue, but merely a light touch used to identify and assess the strength of movement (Griffin, 1974). The patient should then be asked to follow the sequence and swallow the material positioned in his or her mouth. As the patient swallows, the clinician's fingers on the patient's neck can assess initiation of tongue movement on the basis of movement felt by the index finger at the submandibular area immediately behind the anterior mandible. The second finger can perceive hyoid bone movement, and the third and fourth fingers can define laryngeal movement when the swallowing reflex triggers. Comparing the time elapsed between initiation of tongue movement and initiation of hyoid and laryngeal movement can provide the clinician with a very rough estimate of oral transit time, or the time taken from initiation of the swallow by the tongue until the swallowing reflex triggers. The major limitation to this technique is that if the reflex does not trigger in a normal length of time (less than 1 second), the clinician at the bedside cannot assess what is occurring physiologically during the time delay. Movement of the bolus into the pharynx or into the airway cannot be assessed. Thus, only a very gross estimate of oral transit time can be identified, and no real information on the pharyngeal stage of the swallow can be collected.

It is often helpful in assessing aspiration if the patient is asked to perform several additional tasks after the swallow. First, immediately after the swallow the patient should be asked to phonate *ah* for several seconds. The swallowing therapist can then examine the vocal quality for any signs of "gargling," indicative of material sitting on the vocal cords. Immediately after the vocalization, the patient should be asked to pant for

FIGURE 4-15
Positioning of the fingers during the clinical, "bedside," swallowing examination.

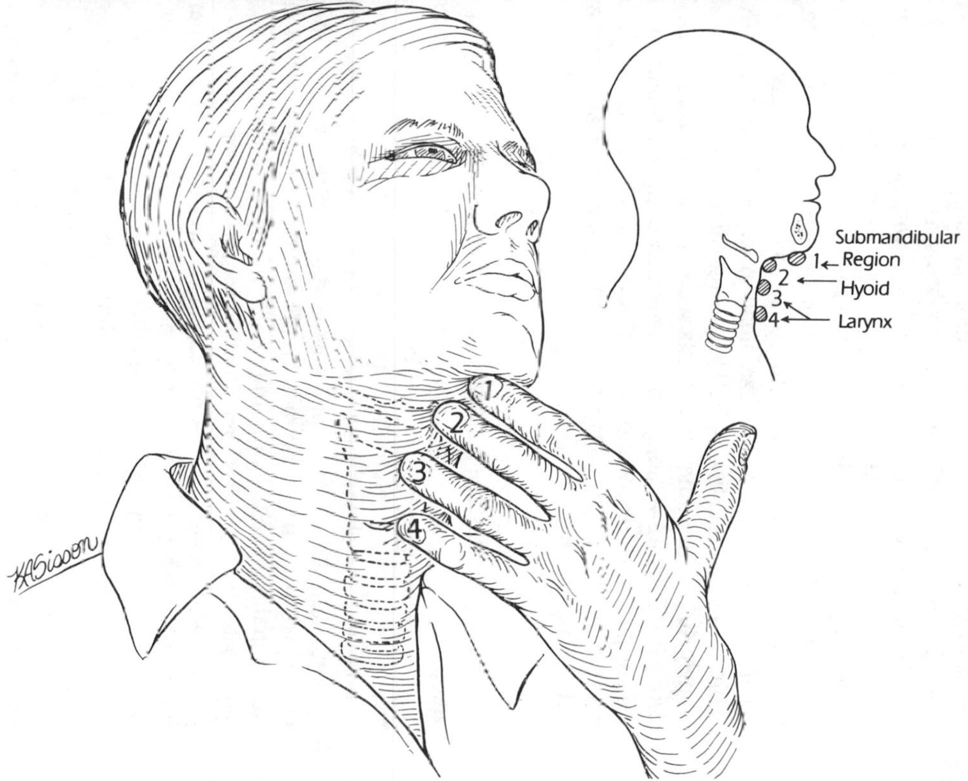

several seconds. In this way, if material is residing in the pharyngeal recesses (valleculae or pyriform sinuses), it will be shaken loose and tend to fall into the airway. After panting, the patient should be asked to vocalize again and vocal quality again evaluated. If the patient coughs during any part of this sequence and expectorates any material or if gargling vocal quality is heard, aspiration can definitely be identified. However, many patients are silent aspirators. That is, they aspirate material past the true vocal cords into the airway without responding in any of the usual ways such as coughing. Thus, the clinician has no way of examining aspiration definitively at the bedside. If a patient aspirates and does not cough or give visible symptoms of aspiration, the clinician will be unaware of entry of material into the airway. A preliminary study of the accuracy of bedside clinical examination of swallowing indicated that clinicians do not identify aspiration during clinical examinations approximately 40% of the time for patients who are actually aspirating. This is strong evidence for a radiographic approach to the examination of swallowing and the assessment of pharyngeal physiology during deglutition in order to identify patients who are aspirating, and the reason and amount of their aspiration.

If videofluoroscopy is not available, still radiographs taken in the lateral planes may be able to provide some information (Sloan, Rickett, Brummett, Bench, & Westover, 1976). The procedure for taking lateral radiographs should be based upon the time frame of normal swallowing. That is, the still radiograph should be taken 2 seconds after the command to swallow has been given to the patient. At this point in time, if swallowing is normal, there should be no residue of material in the oral cavity or pharynx, and the oral and pharyngeal stages of the swallow should be completed. Thus, if the still radiograph shows a large amount of material resting in the valleculae or in the pyriform sinuses or coating the pharyngeal walls, the clinician can identify some degree of disorder in the pharynx and localize it to some extent. However, this is a rather gross judgment which can only point toward the type of dysfunction involved rather than providing an accurate differential diagnosis. Still radiographs can also be taken in the anterior/posterior plane in order to assess asymmetries in collection of material in the valleculae or pyriform sinuses. If vocal cord adduction is to be studied, the patient should be asked to prolong a vowel phonation for several seconds while the radiograph is taken.

When the radiographic or bedside examination has identified the nature of the swallowing disorder or disorders, several management decisions must be made. How should nutrition be managed? If oral feeding is appropriate, what food consistencies should be used? What is the nature of swallowing therapy? Answers to these management questions are based on data collected in the swallowing evaluation and will be discussed in Chapter 5.

Bibliography

Ardran, G., & Kemp, F.   The mechanism of swallowing. *Proceedings of the Royal Society of Medicine,* 1951, *44,* 1038–1040.

Bachman, A.   Methodology in the radiographic examination of the larynx and hypopharynx. *New York State Journal of Medicine,* 1963, *63,* 1155–1163.

Betts, R.   Post-tracheostomy aspiration. *New England Journal of Medicine,* 1965, *273,* 155.

Bonanno, P.   Swallowing dysfunction after tracheostomy. *Annals of Surgery,* 1971, *174,* 29–33.

DeJong, R.   *The neurologic examination.* New York: Hoeber Medical Division—Harper & Row, 1967.

Dobie, R.   Rehabilitation of swallowing disorders. *American Family Physician,* 1978, *27,* 84–95.

Donald, A., & Dawes, J.   A case of dysphagia. *British Medical Journal,* 1977, *30,* 1139–1141.

Edwards, D.   Flow charts, diagnostic keys, and algorithms in the diagnosis of dysphagia. *Scottish Medical Journal,* 1970, *15,* 378–385.

Feldman, S., Deal, C., & Urquhart, W.   Disturbance of swallowing after tracheostomy. *Lancet,* 1966, *1,* 954–955.

Griffin, J., & Tollison, J.   Dysphagia. *American Family Physician,* 1980, *22,* 154–160.

Griffin, K.   Swallowing training for dysphagic patients. *Archives of Physical Medicine and Rehabilitation,* 1974, *55,* 467–470.

Haubrich, W.   In defense of the radiographic diagnosis of dysphagia. *Gastrointestinal Endoscopy,* 1977, *23,* 214.

Kelley, M.   Evaluation of the patient with dysphagia. *Modern Treatment,* 1970, *7,* 1087–1097.

Kirchner, J.   Pharyngeal and esophageal dysfunction: The diagnosis. *Minnesota Medicine,* 1967, *50,* 921–924.

Linden, P., & Siebens, A.   Videofluoroscopy: Use in evaluation and treatment of dysphagia. A miniseminar presented at the American Speech Hearing Language Association annual meeting in Detroit, Nov. 1980.

Maguire, G.   The larynx: Simplified radiological examination using heavy filtration and high voltage. *Radiology,* 1966, *87,* 102–110.

Mandelstam, P., & Lieber, A. Cineradiographic evaluation of the esophagus in normal adults. *Gastroenterology, 1970, 58,* 32–38.

McConchie, I. Dysphagia: General principles of management. *Australian New Zealand Journal of Surgery,* 1973, *42,* 358–359.

Miller, D., & Sethl, G. Tracheal stenosis following prolonged cuffed intubation: Cause and prevention. *Annals of Surgery,* 1970, *171,* 283–293.

Newman, L., Dodaro, R., & Welch, M. A comprehensive program for dysphagia rehabilitation. A workshop conducted at Mercy Hospital and Medical Center, Chicago, May 29, 1980.

O'Connor, A., & Ardran, G. Cinefluorography in the diagnosis of pharyngeal palsies. *Journal of Laryngology and Otology,* 1976, *90,* 1015–1019.

Paloschi, G., & Lynn, R. Observations upon elective and emergency tracheostomy. *Surgery, Gynecology and Obstetrics,* 1965, *120,* 356–358.

Phillips, M., & Hendrix, T. Dysphagia. *Postgraduate Medicine,* 1971, *50,* 81–86.

Pinkus, N. The dangers of oral feeding in the presence of cuffed tracheostomy tubes. *Medical Journal of Australia,* 1973, *1,* 1238–1240.

Pitcher, J. Dysphagia in the elderly: Causes and diagnosis. *Geriatrics,* 1973, *28,* 64–69.

Powers, W., Ogura, J., & Holtz, S. Contrast examination of the larynx and pharynx. *New York State Journal of Medicine,* 1963, *63,* 1163–1173.

Rossato, R., & Wrightson, P., & Donosil, R. Swallow: A test of laryngeal protection. *Surgical Neurology,* 1977, *17,* 24.

Scatliff, J. Cinefluorographic evaluation of the soft tissues of the neck. *New York Journal of Medicine,* 1963, *63,* 1174–1180.

Schultz, A., Niemtzow, P., Jacobs, S., & Naso, F. Dysphagia associated with cricopharyngeal dysfunction. *Archives of Physical Medicine and Rehabilitation,* 1979, *60,* 381–386.

Schuster, M. One swallow does not a diagnosis make. *The American Journal of Medical Sciences,* 1973, *265,* 201–203.

Sellery, G. Airway problems in I.C.U. *International Anesthesiology Clinics,* 1972, *10,* 173–211.

Shahvari, M., Kigin, C., & Zimmerman, J. Speaking tracheostomy tube modified for swallowing dysfunction and chronic aspiration. *Anesthesiology,* 1977, *46,* 290–291.

Shedd, D., Kirchner, J., & Scatliff, J. Oral and pharyngeal components of deglutition. *Archives of Surgery,* 1961, *82,* 373–380.

Sloan, R. Cinefluorographic study of cerebral palsy deglutition. *Journal of the Osaka Dental University,* 1977, *11,* 58–73.

Sloan, R., Ricketts, R., Brummett, S., Bench, R., & Westover, J. Quantified cinefluorographic techniques used in oral roentgenology. *Oral Surgery,* 1965, *20,* 456–463.

Spoerel, W. The unprotected airway. *International Anesthesiology Clinics,* 1972, *10,* 1–35.

Weathers, R., Becker, M., & Genieser, N. Improved technique for study of swallowing function in infants. *Radiologic Technology,* 1974, *46,* 98–100.

5

Management of the Patient with Disordered Oral Feeding

Management Decisions

Two questions to be answered after evaluation of the patient with a problem feeding orally are: what type of nutritional management is necessary; and should therapy include direct or indirect work on swallowing? The continuous goal of any treatment program is the re-establishment of oral feeding while constantly maintaining adequate nutrition. (Aguilar, Olson, & Shedd, 1979; American Dietetic Association, 1980.)

Oral vs.
Non-Oral Feeding

Should the patient continue to be fed orally, or should the patient be placed on a nasogastric tube or given a gastrostomy? At this time, there are no absolute guidelines the clinician can use to make this decision. The results of several studies may be helpful however. In 1979, Logemann, Wheeler, and Sisson examined the relationship between speed of swallowing and diet choices. Patients studied were those with oral cancer who had been treated surgically, and who were provided with an oral prosthesis to assist in eating and talking. Patients were studied over a 6-month period, and careful records were kept regarding diet choices, amount of food eaten, and speed of eating. Measures of oral and pharyngeal transit time taken at 1-, 2-, 3- and 6-month intervals were compared with the food consistencies actually included in the patient's diet. These data are shown in Figure 5-1. Examination of these data reveals that patients do

129

FIGURE 5-1
Combined oral and pharyngeal transit times for surgically treated oral cancer patients for paste consistency foods, and notation of whether patients included paste consistency foods in their daily diet.

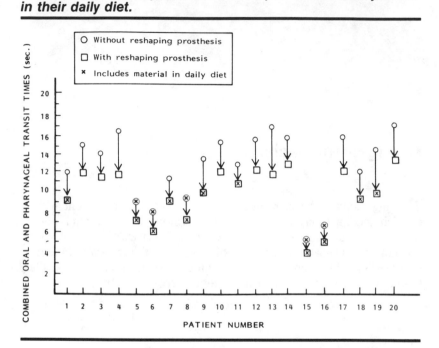

not include a particular food consistency in their diet unless the combined oral and pharyngeal transit time for swallow of that material is approximately 10 seconds or less. These data corroborate earlier patient reports. When it takes a long time to eat a particular food consistency, i.e. more than 10 seconds, patients will discontinue eating that consistency of food or will not get a sufficient amount of food down to maintain their weight.

Thus, *time* taken to swallow a single bolus of a particular consistency of food appears to be an important parameter in nutritional management. If the radiographic study indicates that it takes the patient more than 10 seconds to eat *every* consistency of food tried, the patient may feed by mouth but will need a nasogastric tube to supplement oral feedings and to provide adequate nutrition. If the swallowing therapist indicates that the patient's progress in therapy is slow, and it appears that it will take more than 3 months to improve the patient's swallowing to the point that he or she will not need the supplemental feedings, the managing physician may

FIGURE 5-2
Percent aspiration on liquid swallows for surgically treated oral cancer patients, and notation of whether patients included liquids in their daily diet.

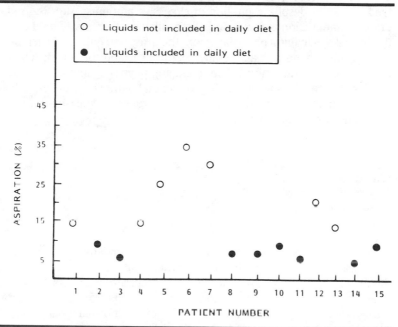

prefer to give the patient a gastrostomy rather than leave the nasogastric tube in place for that long a period. Some physicians do not like to leave a nasogastric tube in place for more than 3 to 4 weeks. Or, the patient may be taught to place the nasogastric tube at each meal and remove it after feeding.

In some cases, if the patient's function is borderline, i.e. approximately 10 seconds, the dietitian may provide the patient with diet supplements to increase the caloric content of the foods eaten orally.

A second parameter of swallowing function that these authors (Logemann, Wheeler, & Sisson, 1979) examined in relation to diet choices was *aspiration.* The gross approximation of amount of material aspirated was correlated with selection of diet choices by the patient. All of these patients were aware of their aspiration. These data are shown in Figure 5-2. It is clear that if patients aspirate any more than 10% of each bolus, and they are aware of that aspiration, they will eliminate that food consistency from their diet. These data indicate that if a patient is unable to swallow any food consistency with less than 10% aspiration, he or she will stop eating. However, those patients who are unaware of their swallowing disorder, particularly the neurologic group, will persevere in attempting to feed by mouth despite aspiration of excessive amounts. After the radiographic examination is completed, the swallowing therapist should inform the patient's managing physician about the gross percentage of each bolus that is aspirated, despite all therapy attempts (e.g. posture change, voluntarily protecting the airway). The managing physician should then make the decision regarding oral feeding. In general, however, a patient who is aspirating more than 10% of every bolus, regardless of consistency of food, should not be feeding orally.

Direct vs. Indirect Therapy for the Swallowing Disorder

The second decision in management of the patient with disordered feeding is whether to work directly on swallowing—to introduce food into the mouth and attempt to reinforce the appropriate behaviors during the swallow—or to work indirectly on swallowing, using exercises to improve those motor controls that are prerequisites for normal swallowing. In general, this decision is made based on the information on aspiration gained from the radiographic study. Typically, this information should be provided to the patient's physician and he or she should decide whether the patient can tolerate aspiration of the designated amount. In general, if the patient is aspirating more than 10% of each bolus swallowed and therapeutic techniques applied at the time are unable to reduce this aspiration, the patient will function better if therapy focuses on improving the muscle controls required for the swallowing rather than working directly on swallowing by using food or liquid (Griffin, 1974). It is of no help to place the patient in a situation where he or she is continuously aspirating with no hope of deterring material from entering the airway during the swallowing regimen.

Only the radiographic study can provide the data necessary to make these decisions. Aspiration can be clearly observed only during the radiographic study. The clinician working on swallowing without benefit of data from a radiographic study is likely to make a number of erroneous management decisions.

Therapy Techniques

Indirect Therapy

Indirect therapy for swallowing disorders generally involves one of three types of exercises: (1) exercises to improve oral motor control of the bolus and the voluntary stage of the swallow (Aguilar et al., 1979); (2) stimulation of the swallowing reflex to heighten the reflex when a swallow is attempted; and, (3) exercises to increase adduction of tissues at the top of the airway usually the true vocal folds, to improve airway protection during the swallow.

Oral Motor Control Exercises

Most frequently patients have difficulty with six aspects of tongue control during swallowing: (1) lateralization of the tongue during chewing, (2) elevation of the tongue to the hard palate, (3) cupping of the tongue around the bolus to hold it in a cohesive manner, (4) elevation of the tongue against the palate to hold the bolus, (5) *range* of anterior to posterior movement of the tongue in the initiation of the voluntary or oral stage of the swallow, and (6) *organized* anterior to posterior tongue movement to initiate the swallow. The exercises given below cover each of these six goals. In all cases, directions for exercise regimens should be written down for the patient so that he or she can repeat them without the therapist present.

Range of Tongue Motion Exercises. Exercises to increase range of tongue motion, including tongue elevation and lateralization, should improve oral transit. The patient should be asked to open his or her mouth as wide as possible and elevate the tongue as high as possible in the front, to hold it there for 1 second, and to release it. Then the patient should elevate the back of the tongue as far as possible, hold it there for 1 second, and release it. This procedure should continue with the patient stretching the tongue to each side as far as possible, extending the tongue out of his or her mouth as far as possible, and pulling it back as far as possible, holding for 1 second in each direction. This entire series of range of motion exercises should be repeated 5 to 10 times in one session so the exercise lasts approximately 3 or 4 minutes. The entire set of exercises should be repeated 5 to 10 times a day.

Resistance Exercises. Pushing the tongue against a tongue blade, popsicle, sucker, or the clinician's finger will improve both range of motion and strength (Jordan, 1979). The patient can be asked to push his or her tongue *up* against the tongue blade, to the side against the tongue blade, or thrust forward against it. In each case the patient should hold the pressure against the tongue blade for 1 second, and the tongue blade should be held at the point of the patient's maximum range of movement in each direction.

Bolus Control Exercises. A number of exercises can be used to improve lingual control of the bolus without asking the patient to swallow.

Exercises To Improve Gross Manipulation of Material. The patient should be given something large to manipulate in the mouth which can be controlled by the clinician, such as a flexible licorice whip. The patient can manipulate one end of the licorice with the tongue while the clinician holds the other end, thereby preventing patient loss of control and choking. At first, the patient is asked simply to grasp the licorice stick between the tongue and palate, to move it from one side to the other and to slide it forward and backward. After each attempt, the patient should be asked to judge the success of the attempt and to identify where the material is in the mouth. When the patient is able to move the licorice in a gross way, he or she should be asked to move it in a circular fashion from the middle of the mouth to the teeth on one side, back to the middle of the mouth and back to the teeth on the same side, in the way that the tongue manipulates food during chewing. When the patient is able to make these movements with some speed (approximately three directions in 1 second), he or she should be asked to repeat the same motions with a lifesaver tied to a thread held by the clinician, and then with a thin cloth tape soaked in a small amount of orange juice or cranberry juice (only if aspiration is minimal). This last provides the patient with some taste, a very small amount of liquid to swallow, and a smaller object (still controlled by the clinician) to manipulate in the mouth. When control improves, the patient is given chewing gum that must be manipulated without the clinician's control (Ford, Grotz, Pomerantz, Bruno, & Flannery, 1974).

In addition to manipulating material from side-to-side in the mouth without losing control of it, the patient needs to be able to hold both a liquid and paste bolus in a cohesive fashion.

Exercises To Hold a Cohesive Bolus. This exercise should be started only when the patient has demonstrated the ability to manipulate material grossly in the mouth, as described in the previous exercise. It is usually easiest to begin with a paste consistency bolus, approximately ⅓ of a teaspoon. The bolus is placed on the patient's tongue and he or she is asked to move the bolus around the mouth, without losing the material or allowing it to spread out around the mouth. This requires that the patient cup the tongue around the bolus. When the patient is finished, the bolus can be expectorated rather than swallowed, and the clinician can examine the patient's mouth for any residue. When the patient is successful at this task, the paste bolus can be varied in size, repeating the same procedure.

Then a liquid bolus can be used. Liquid, ⅓ teaspoon, can be placed in the patient's mouth, and the patient asked to keep the liquid together and to move it about the mouth without losing it or swallowing it. When finished, the patient can spit out the material.

Bolus Propulsion Exercises. The patient may also need to practice posterior propulsion of the bolus. This can be accomplished using a long narrow wad of gauze soaked in cranberry or orange juice. With this placed in the mouth the patient can be asked to push upward and backward against the gauze with the tongue, squeezing liquid out of the gauze and pushing it backward at the same time. With the clinician holding the front of the gauze, it cannot be swallowed but can give the patient practice in pushing material upward and backward with the tongue. The small amount of liquid can stimulate a swallow. The amount of liquid placed in the gauze will depend upon the patient's ability to control liquid once it enters the pharyngeal stage of the swallow.

Therapy To Stimulate the Swallowing Reflex

A large number of patients, particularly neurologically impaired patients, exhibit delayed triggering of the swallowing reflex. Triggering of the reflex initiates a number of simultaneous motor acts: elevation of the soft palate to close off the velopharyngeal port, elevation and closure of the larynx to protect the airway, contraction of the pharyngeal constrictors to initiate peristalsis, and finally, as a part of the sequential peristaltic action, relaxation of the cricopharyngeal muscle at the top of the esophagus to allow the bolus to pass easily into the esophagus. If the reflex does not trigger, material coming over the base of the tongue will collect in the recesses of the pharynx, including the valleculae and pyriform sinuses, and/or will splash into the airway, which is standing open until the reflex triggers. In patients whose swallowing reflex does not trigger or triggers late, therapy is designed to stimulate the reflex. The reflex is typically triggered in the faucial arch area, particularly at the base of the anterior faucial arch. To trigger the reflex a small, long-handled laryngeal mirror (#00 or #0—approximately ½" in diameter) is used because it permits the clinician to manipulate the head of the mirror easily in the patient's mouth and to place it with acccuracy at the base of the faucial arches. To stimulate the reflex, the mirror is held in ice water for approximately 10 seconds and then lightly touched to the base of the anterior faucial arch, as shown in Figure 5-3. Light contact is repeated 5 to 10 times. During these repeated contacts, it is unlikely that an actual swallow will be triggered. Rather, the purpose of the exercise is to heighten the sensitivity of the reflex so that when food or liquid *is* presented and the patient attempts a voluntary swallow, the reflex will be triggered. At most the clinician may observe the thyroid cartilage elevate or the faucial arches or soft palate twitch during the actual stimulation.

With a patient whose physician has ordered no oral feeding, the clinician can ask the patient to swallow after the stimulation without presenting any liquid. Then the clinician should carefully observe the swallowing mechanism by placing outstretched fingers lightly on the patient's neck, with the forefinger at the tip of the mandible, second finger on the hyoid bone, and third and fourth fingers on the thyroid cartilage and cricoid cartilages respectively, as discussed in Chapter 3. With the index finger on the tip of the mandible and the second finger on the hyoid, the first lingual movement at the initiation of the posterior propulsion of the bolus (which defines the beginning of the oral transit time) can be felt. When the swallowing reflex is initiated, the larynx elevates and the hyoid bone moves upward and backward. Triggering of the swallowing reflex marks the end of the oral stage of the swallow. Therefore, oral transit time can be measured by the time interval between the initiation of lingual movement and the elevation of the larynx indicating the swallowing reflex has triggered. If oral transit is greater than 1 second it is abnormal.

If the patient can tolerate small amounts of material, the clinician may introduce a small amount of liquid as follows and ask the patient to swallow. After 5 or 10 repeated light contacts of the laryngeal mirror against the faucial arches, a straw can be effectively used as a pipette, filling it with approximately ¼ inch of ice water. The pipette is then placed with its fluid-filled end at the anterior faucial arch, where contact of the laryngeal mirror was made during stimulation. The patient is then instructed to attempt to swallow when the clinician releases the liquid and gives the command, "Now." For added stimulation, iced gingerale or other carbonated beverage may be used rather than ice water. To assure that any liquids swallowed can be detected if expectorated orally or through a tracheostomy site after the swallow, food coloring can be added to the liquid.

FIGURE 5-3
Front view of the oral cavity with a tongue blade holding the right lip out of the way while the #00 laryngeal mirror is positioned for stimulation of the swallowing reflex at the base of the anterior faucial arch.

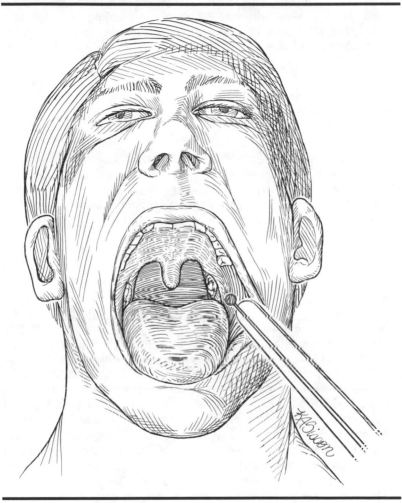

In severely impaired patients, it is likely that no reflex will be triggered with attempts to swallow (with or without liquid) during the early sessions of reflex stimulation. Stimulation will need to be repeated four or five times daily for 5 to 10 minutes each time for several weeks to a month.

Once the swallowing reflex begins to trigger, therapy may be expanded by: (1) increasing, in very small steps, the amount of material presented to the patient in a single swallow (still in the pipette at the base of the faucial arches) and (2) changing the consistency of the food presented at the faucial arches (increasing thickness). The progression of therapy in these patients is often slow, with restoration of oral feeding often taking a number of months. During this time these patients will need a nasogastric tube or gastrostomy to maintain nutrition.

Exercises To Increase Adduction of Tissues at the Top of the Airway

If laryngeal incompetence during swallowing cannot be managed quickly by postural assists or teaching the patient to voluntarily close the airway, a sequence of laryngeal adduction exercises should be initiated prior to any actual swallowing therapy. The patient is asked to complete the series 5 to 10 times daily for 5 minutes each time. Initially, the patient should be seated and told to hold his or her breath as tightly as possible while pushing down or pulling up on the chair with both hands for 5 seconds. Then the patient is asked to bear down against a chair with only one hand (rather than two) and to produce clear voice simultaneously. After repeating this exercise 5 times, the patient is asked to repeat "ah" 5 times with hard glottal attack on each vowel. These 3 exercises are repeated 3 times in a sequence, 5 to 10 times a day. It should be carefully explained that the patient can monitor improvements in laryngeal function by listening to the clarity of voice quality. It should also be explained that the exercises involving lifting, pushing, and vocalization are directly applicable to swallowing as these increase muscle activity in the larynx and are basic to good laryngeal closure during swallowing. The patient should continue to practice this series of exercises for about 1 week. After 1 week of these exercises, if swallowing re-evaluation does not reveal sufficient improvement with the larynx providing good airway protection during swallowing, the exercises should be changed. This is to prevent monotony for the patient more than to provide a hierarchy of difficulty.

The second set of exercises involves lifting or pushing with simultaneous voicing, such as pulling up on a chair with both hands while prolonging phonation. The repeated glottal attack exercise may be made more difficult by asking the patient to begin phonation on "ah" with a hard attack and to sustain the phonation with clear, smooth vocal quality for 5 to 10 seconds. Finally, the patient should be asked to practice a "pseudo" supraglottic swallow—that is to take a breath, hold it, and cough as strongly as possible. In this way the patient practices the adduction/expectoration steps of the supraglottic swallow. These movements may be incorporated into the practice of the entire supraglottic swallow sequence without giving the patient any material to be swallowed. The entire sequence involves taking a breath, holding the breath while swallowing, and releasing the breath into a cough to expectorate any residual material.

In most cases, these exercises will effect improvement within 2 weeks. Occasionally, however, it will take 6 to 8 months for some patients to attain adequate airway protection. Most often these are the patients who have undergone an extended supraglottic laryngectomy.

Direct Therapy To Improve Swallowing Disorders

Direct therapy involves presenting food or liquid to the patient and asking him or her to swallow it while following specified instructions. In some cases, these exercises may involve simply positioning the head a particular way so aspiration is eliminated. In other cases, the sequence of instructions may include as many as seven steps and may only improve his or her swallowing a moderate amount. In all instances, the patient should be given written instructions describing the appropriate steps to follow. The rationale for the procedures should be discussed with the patient and the patient should be given ample time to practice the sequence of instructions on dry swallows before proceeding to swallows of food or liquid (Buckley, Addicks, & Maniglia, 1976; Griffin, 1974).

Whenever food or liquid is provided for practice swallows, only small amounts should be given (Buckley et al., 1976). The amount to be swallowed should be shown to the patient as reassurance that the food or liquid cannot obliterate the airway. The patient should also be encouraged to cough whenever needed to clear the airway. Patients should never be allowed to feel that coughing should be restrained because it is a sign of failure to swallow correctly. Instead, they should be positively reinforced for coughing as needed (Dobie, 1978).

Therapy techniques will be discussed for each of the swallowing disorders described in Chapter 3. The exercises discussed are not meant to be prescriptions nor to be all-inclusive lists. Rather, they are methods that have been found to improve swallowing in a number of patients with each disorder. It is likely there are other procedures not included here that would also improve the patient's swallowing. The techniques discussed here are summarized in Table 5-1.

TABLE 5-1.
Therapy Techniques for Swallowing Problems.

SWALLOWING DISTURBANCE– PHYSIOLOGIC	*THERAPY*
Oral stage of the swallow	
Reduction in lip closure	Lip exercises
Reduction in cheek tension	Posture (tilt toward stronger side) Pressure on weaker side
Reduction in tongue elevation	Tongue exercises Position food posteriorly Prosthesis Posture (tilt head backward)
Reduced tongue lateralization, anterior to posterior movement	Prosthesis Tongue exercises Position food posteriorly Posture (tilt head backward)
Reflex	
Delayed or absent reflex	Thermal stimulation Posture (tilt head forward)
Pharyngeal stage of the swallow	
Reduced pharyngeal peristalsis	Alternate liquid/solid swallows
Pharyngeal hemiparesis	Posture (tilt toward stronger side, turn toward weaker side)
Reduced laryngeal elevation	Supraglottic swallow
Reduced laryngeal closure	Adduction exercises Supraglottic swallow
Cricopharyngeal hypertonicity	Myotomy
SWALLOWING DISTURBANCES –ANATOMIC	
Tongue scarring	Surgical release Position of food
Cervical osteophyte	Surgical removal Diet change
Scar tissue on pharyngeal wall	Posture
Scar tissue at base of tongue	Surgical removal
Tracheo-esophageal fistula	Surgical closure
Zenker's diverticulum	Surgical removal

Posture changes are suggested as therapy techniques for a number of types of dysphagic patients. Though some authors recommend a single posture for optimum swallowing (generally with the head tilted forward at a 45° angle (Buckley et al., 1976; Gaffney & Campbell, 1974; Larsen, 1973), there is no single posture which improves swallowing in all patients. Rather, there are a variety of postural changes that will improve specific swallowing disorders. The swallowing therapist must first correctly diagnose the physiological or anatomic disorder in the patient's deglutition and then identify the posture which will facilitate most normal swallowing.

Disorders Affecting Mastication

As a temporary measure, the patient with difficulty chewing may restrict his diet to liquids and soft foods while working on mastication.

Reduced Range of Tongue Movement Laterally. Exercises to improve range of lateral tongue movement have been described earlier in the section on indirect swallowing therapy procedures. As a temporary measure, the patient whose tongue elevation is normal may be taught to mash food by pressing the tongue against the roof of the mouth. Or, the patient may position food on the most mobile side of the tongue (Buckley et al., 1976).

Reduced Buccal Tension/Buccal Scarring. To improve buccal tension, the patient may be given facial exercises. These include rounding the lips tightly for "oh" and stretching the lips broadly for "ee." Rapidly alternating these two postures may increase buccal tension. Also, smiling broadly and spreading the lips tightly across the teeth may also improve cheek tension.

In the interim, the patient may be taught to place external pressure on the affected cheek and thus close the sulcus between the cheek and the lower alveolus. Gently resting one hand against the affected cheek should provide sufficient pressure.

Placing food on the unaffected side and tilting the head towards the unaffected side may also be helpful, as it will keep food on the stronger side (Buckley et al., 1976).

Reduced Range of Mandibular Movement Laterally. The patient may be given mandibular range of motion exercises. These exercises involve opening the jaw as widely as possible and holding the maximum opening for 1 second; opening and moving the jaw to each side as far as possible and holding the extended position in each direction for 1 second; and moving the jaw around in a circle as far as possible in each direction. Occasionally, the clinician may assist the patient's attempts at jaw movement by placing external pressure on the mandible in the desired direction of movement. The patient should always be instructed to move the jaw as far as possible in each direction, feeling a strong pull but no pain. If any pain occurs, the exercise should be discontinued until the patient can talk with the swallowing therapist or the doctor. This kind of exercise is particularly important for postoperative oral cancer patients, as they may experience some scarring of the muscles of mastication. The exercises should also be continued through radiotherapy and for 6 to 8 weeks after radiation therapy, as radiotherapy may increase the fibrosis in the muscles of mastication.

If the patient is completely unable to lateralize the mandible and thus get normal occlusion, the individual may be taught to mash food with the tongue against the palate in order to broaden diet options.

In some cases a guide plane prosthesis is helpful. Such a prosthesis involves a vertical bar attached to a lower denture or partial. When the patient closes his or her mouth, the vertical bar guides the mandible into proper alignment, and thus proper occlusion.

Reduced Range of Tongue Movement Vertically. Exercises for this problem have been described in the section on indirect therapy for swallowing. If, however, the patient has not achieved a tongue-to-palate contact after several months of repeating these exercises at regular intervals, a palate reshaping prosthesis may be given (Logemann, Sisson, & Wheeler, 1980; Wheeler, Logemann, & Rosen, 1980; Trible, 1967). If such a prosthesis is made and the patient's tongue elevation continues to improve, the palate can be reshaped with some of the bulk removed to allow for this improved tongue movement.

The speech pathologist and maxillofacial prosthodontist work together to construct the prosthesis, which is designed to lower the palatal vault to complement tongue function. Several prostheses are illustrated in Figure 5-4a-d. If a patient has generalized reduction in tongue elevation both anteriorly and posteriorly, the palate would be lowered uniformly. If the patient exhibits a hemiparesis or has lost one longitudinal half of the tongue in ablative surgery, the prosthesis would contain more material on the affected side.

The ultimate design of the prosthesis will depend on speech needs as well as swallowing patterns, so the final configuration may be a compromise between the optimum shape for the two functions.

FIGURE 5-4 (a-d)
Frontal (c and d) and lateral (a and b) views of intra-oral palatal reshaping prostheses designed to lower the palatal arch and facilitate tongue to palate contact.

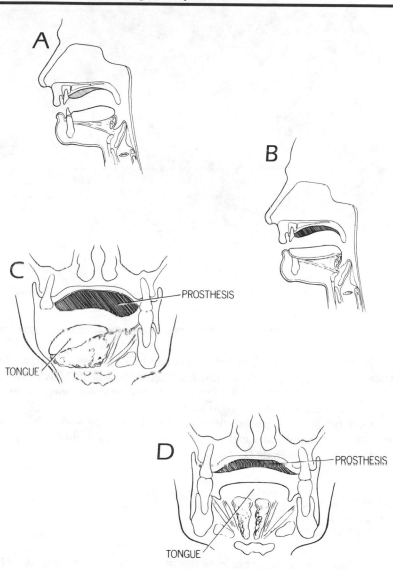

FIGURE 5-5
A palatal reshaping prosthesis with wire clasps to fit around the patient's existing upper teeth.

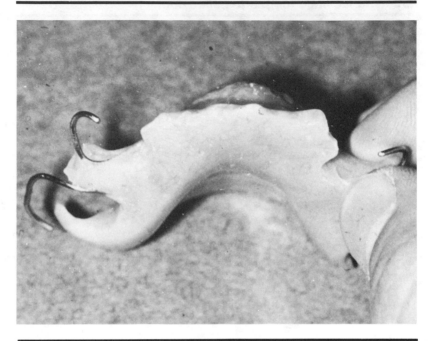

The prosthesis may contain no teeth and be designed to clasp to the patient's existing dentition, as shown in Figure 5-5; it may have several teeth to replace missing dental units; or it may be constructed as a full upper denture, as shown in Figure 5-6.

Other types of prostheses, such as mandibular tongue prostheses to improve the patient's oral manipulation of food and speed of oral transit may also be considered (Leonard & Gillis, 1982).

**Disorders Affecting the
Preparatory Phase
of the Swallow**

During the preparatory phase of the swallow, the patient must be able to manipulate food in the mouth while maintaining complete closure of

FIGURE 5-6
A palatal reshaping prosthesis constructed as part of a full upper denture.

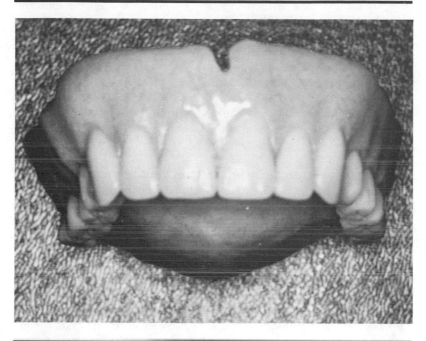

the lips—while controlling the bolus so that nothing spills into the pharynx.

Reduced Labial Closure. To improve labial closure, range of lip motion exercises may be necessary first. These exercises include: (1) stretching the lips in the /i/ position as far as possible and holding for one second; (2) puckering the lips as tightly as possible and holding for 1 second; and, (3) bringing the lips together and holding tightly for 1 second. If lip closure is not possible on the third exercise, the patient can close his or her lips against a spoon or other object. As strength and range of motion improve, the size of the object can be reduced until it is only the thickness of a tongue blade, and closure can be obtained. Once the patient is able to obtain lip closure, but has not habituated it, a graduated increase in the time required to maintain closure should be used. The patient may be asked to hold lip closure for 1 minute. This should be repeated 10 times a day. The next day the patient should maintain lip closure for 2 minutes, 10 times a day. The schedule should be increased 1 minute a day until the patient reaches 10 minutes per time. After 2 weeks of following the regimen regularly, the patient should have habituated normal lip closure. Mitchell (1967) described a buccinator apparatus to remind the patient to keep the mouth closed until closure can be accomplished automatically. The device consisted of flat-shaped #16 gauge indoor-outdoor wire, cut to the length which encircles the patient's lips. The overlapped ends are wrapped with tape and positioned on the outside of the lower lip at the base of the lower teeth. The author states, "By contouring the wire around the buccinator muscle and by applying pressure at the base of the nose and at the base of the lower teeth, the device pulls the lips in and holds the teeth together" (p. 1135).

Closing the lips against resistance both laterally and anteriorly, may help to improve lip closure. Using a tongue blade, the patient can be asked to close the lips tightly around the tongue blade and hold it with the lips while the patient or the clinician attempts to extract it. This exercise will also increase lip strength.

Another such exercise involves maintaining lip closure while the patient or the clinician tries to manually part the lips.

Reduced Tongue Movement To Form the Bolus. Exercises to improve tongue movement in formation of the bolus are discussed in the section on indirect swallowing procedures. However as an interim measure, the clinician may suggest that the patient tilt his or her head slightly forward to keep the bolus in the anterior part of the mouth until the patient is ready to initiate the swallow, thus preventing him or her from losing it in one of the lateral sulci. With the start of the swallow, the patient may then change head posture as appropriate.

Reduced Range and Coordination of Tongue Movement to Hold the Bolus. Exercises for range and coordination of tongue movement in controlling the bolus are discussed in the section on indirect therapy techniques for swallowing. As an interim measure, the clinician may suggest that the patient not attempt to manipulate the bolus once it is in the mouth but to hold the material securely against the front of the roof of the mouth and to initiate the swallow immediately.

In addition, the patient may hold his or her head slightly downward to keep the bolus in the more anterior position.

Reduced Ability To Hold the Bolus in Normal Position. The patient may be given a bolus of paste consistency (approximately ⅓ teaspoon) and asked to hold it consciously against the anterior to mid portion of the palate with the tongue. This exercise requires that the tongue tip be contacting the alveolar ridge immediately posterior to the teeth.

Reduced Oral Sensitivity. The patient with reduced oral sensitivity should position food on the more sensitive side of his or her oral cavity. In addition, the use of cold liquid may help the individual to localize the material in the mouth. The use of mild spices or tastes to which the patient is sensitive may also improve his or her localization of material in the mouth.

Disorders Affecting the
Oral Phase of the Swallow

A number of techniques may be employed to improve the oral phase of the swallow. Some of these are compensatory in nature—that is, they are not designed to improve function, but are designed to allow the patient to compensate for his or her problem. Others are rehabilitative in nature— designed to help the patient reclaim normal movement patterns.

Tongue Thrust. In tongue thrust, the patient pushes the tongue an- teriorly against the central incisors to initiate the swallow. This volume will not address the problem of developmental tongue thrust, which is a complicated one, requiring more attention than is given here. The em- phasis here is on the neurologically impaired patient who acquires a tongue thrust as a result of a neurologic lesion. In these patients, height- ening their awareness of the thrust pattern and asking them to con- sciously position their tongue on the alveolar ridge and begin the swallow with an upward-backward push will often reduce the thrusting.

As a compensatory measure, the patient may be taught to position food posteriorly on the tongue and thus avoid the thrusting pattern. In some instances, the tongue thrust is severe enough to actually throw material from the mouth.

Reduced Tongue Elevation. Exercises to improve tongue elevation have been discussed in the section on indirect exercises to improve swallowing. As an interim measure, the patient may be taught to position food posteriorly in the oral cavity or to syringe liquid into the oral pharynx and bypass the necessity of tongue elevation (Buckley et al. 1976; Trible, 1967). If the patient is able to suck, positioning a straw far posteriorly in the oral cavity almost at the level of the faucial arches may facilitate liquid swallows.

The patient may also be taught to tilt the head backward to allow gravity to assist in propelling food from the oral cavity into the pharynx (Trible, 1967). This technique will not increase the patient's chances of aspiration if the patient has a normal swallow reflex and normal laryngeal control. If the clinician is concerned that the patient may aspirate because of the rapidity with which food is thrust into the pharynx, the clinician may teach the patient to voluntarily protect his or her airway using the supraglottic swallow technique. In this technique, the patient is taught to take a breath and hold it during the swallow (Larsen, 1973). In the case of the individual with reduced tongue elevation the patient's swallowing sequence may be: First take a breath and hold it, then place the food in the mouth, then tilt the head backward and swallow, then cough after the swallow to rid the pharynx of any residue of material. In this sequence voluntarily closing the airway prevents any aspiration that may occur before the swallowing reflex is triggered.

Reduced Anterior to Posterior Tongue Movement. Exercises to improve range of anterior to posterior tongue movement are discussed in the section on techniques for indirectly working on swallowing.

Again, the same compensatory postures and positions of food in the oral cavity described in the section on exercises to improve tongue elevation may be used for patients with reduced anterior to posterior tongue movement. Frequently, the same patients experience reduced tongue range of motion in both elevation and anterior to posterior movement.

Disorganized Anterior to Posterior Tongue Movement. Some types of patients exhibit specific patterns of tongue movement that are severely disorganized and result in long delays in oral transit. Parkinsonian patients are such a group. They exhibit a rapidly repeating tongue pumping action that keeps food in the oral cavity for long periods of time. One way to reduce this activity is to alert the patient to the pumping, and ask him or her to consciously hold the bolus against the palate with the tongue and to initiate the swallow with a single strong backward movement of the tongue. This will normally eliminate or reduce the disorganized tongue pattern as long as the patient can remain aware of his or her swallowing pattern.

Scarred Tongue Contour. A scarred tongue contour cannot be improved with exercises. It may be compensated for by teaching the patient to position food posterior to this scarring, and to tilt the head backward to use gravity to assist in oral transit. Actual treatment for the scarring involves surgical release of the scar, and the patient should be referred to the head and neck surgeon for corrective measures. In many cases, it is necessary to show the patient's videofluoroscopic study, which has been recorded on videotape, to the head and neck surgeon in order for the physician to appreciate the seriousness of the disorder as it impacts on swallowing. The effect of scarring is usually not seen except in the dynamics of movement. If the head and neck surgeon simply examines the patient's oral cavity at rest, the scar may seem rather small and insignificant. However, during tongue movement for swallowing, when the anterior and posterior tongue segments elevate and the scar tissue does not, a large depression is created into which most or all of the bolus of food collects. The patient is thus unable to move food posteriorly.

Disorders Affecting
the Pharyngeal Stage
of the Swallow

Disorders affecting the pharyngeal stage of the swallow will have been diagnosed from videofluoroscopic studies.

Delayed or Absent Swallowing Reflex. Treatment for a delayed or absent swallowing reflex involves stimulation of the reflex, as described earlier in this chapter under techniques to improve swallowing indirectly. This stimulation usually needs to be repeated 3 times a day for 5 to 10 minutes each time. The patient or a family member may be taught to do this stimulation when the patient leaves the hospital.

One technique to compensate for delayed swallowing reflex is to ask the patient to tilt the head forward when swallowing. Tilting the head forward widens the vallecular space and increases the chance that the bolus will hesitate in the valleculae prior to the triggering of the reflex, rather than falling into the airway. Patients with delayed or absent swallowing reflex should also limit the amount of each bolus so the bolus can be held in the pharyngeal recesses and the mass is not so large that it will overflow into the open airway.

The speed at which the patient swallows is also an important factor. Once the radiographic study has determined the time for the delay in the reflex, the patient and his or her family should be warned that the patient needs this amount of time between swallows to insure that each bolus has cleared the pharynx before a new swallow is initiated. Otherwise, the patient will overflow his or her pharyngeal recesses and aspirate significantly.

Heimlich and O'Connor (1979a, 1979b) described an unusual technique employed with three patients who had "forgotten" how to swallow. The procedure involved 4 sequential steps. First, the patient placed one gloved index finger in the instructor's mouth and the other hand against the upper throat and chin of the instructor so the patient could experience the sensation of the instructor sucking the finger while feeling the swallowing movements in the therapist's neck. Second, the patient put a finger into his or her own mouth, trying to imitate the sucking sensation, and placed the other hand on his or her own upper neck to attempt to duplicate the swallowing process. Third, a specially designed plastic tube (the Mackler type) was placed in the cervical esophagus with its flared end above the cricopharyngeus, allowing free access of saliva into the upper esophagus, and the patient repeated the sucking and swallowing process. And, fourth, when the ability to swallow liquids was mastered with the tube, the tube was removed and instruction continued until a normal diet was resumed. Care was taken not to perforate the esophagus with the tube and not to allow displacement of the prosthesis upward or downward.

Reduced Pharyngeal Peristalsis. There is no direct therapy technique to improve pharyngeal peristalsis. Compensatory techniques include: (1) alternating liquid and semisolid or solid swallows so the liquid washes the material of thicker consistency through the pharynx; (2) limiting the diet to liquids or thin paste materials requiring less peristaltic action to clear the pharynx; and (3) following each swallow of food or liquid with several repetitive "dry" swallows to clear the pharynx of any residual material.

In some cases, teaching the patient a supraglottic swallow or voluntary airway protection may be helpful. The patient's expectoration would clear the residual material from the pharynx.

Unilateral Pharyngeal Paralysis. There is no exercise which will improve pharyngeal paralysis. However, there are a number of compensatory techniques.

The patient may be taught to *turn* his or her head toward the *affected* side, thus closing the pyriform sinus on the affected side and directing material down the more normal side (Kirchner, 1967).

Or, if the patient has a unilateral paralysis in lingual function as well as the pharynx, the patient may function better by *tilting* the head toward the *stronger* side, thus keeping material on the stronger side in the oral cavity as well as through the pharynx.

Additionally, the patient may be taught the supraglottic swallow in order to expectorate any residual material that remains in the pharynx. Or the patient may alternate liquid and solid swallows in order to wash away thicker food that remains in the pharynx after the swallow.

Cervical Osteophyte. A cervical osteophyte, or boney overgrowth of one of the cervical vertebra, must be surgically reduced, or the patient may acclimate to it by thinning out the consistency of material swallowed. Foods of a thicker consistency will be more difficult.

Scarred Pharyngeal Wall. The same techniques that improve or compensate for unilateral pharyngeal paralysis may be used for a scarred pharyngeal wall. The scarring often collects material which will remain at the scar site after the swallow, so that the supraglottic swallow sequence may help to eliminate this residue.

Scar Tissue at the Base of the Tongue. Many total laryngectomees who have been closed with vertical closure will develop a scar tissue ledge from the side of the pharynx which, on lateral radiography, appears to be an epiglottis. When the patient attempts to swallow, this scar tissue widens with the pull of the pharyngeal constrictors and acts as a side pocket in the pharynx. This scar tissue band can be surgically removed, or the patient can adjust to it by swallowing only liquids and thin paste consistencies.

Cricopharyngeal Dysfunction. There are no exercises that will improve cricopharyngeal dysfunction except those described by Schultz, Niemtzow, Jacobs, and Naso (1979). These investigators studied three patients after cricopharyngeal dysfunction and long periods of therapy involving the establishment of voluntary control of the cricopharyngeus, similar to that learned by total laryngectomees to take air in for esophageal voice. The investigators were able to ameliorate the dysfunction but only after a number of months. The more usual treatment for cricopharyngeal dysfunction is dilatation (a temporary solution), or a cricopharyngeal myotomy to slit the muscle. These techniques are discussed in Chapter 9.

Reduced Laryngeal Elevation. A technique to compensate for reduced laryngeal elevation involves teaching the patient the supraglottic swallow. This technique is helpful because the patient will expectorate the residual material left above the larynx after the swallow. Thus, aspiration after the swallow is minimized. In some cases, the patient does not need to learn the entire supraglottic sequence, but instead can be taught to simply clear the throat immediately after the swallow and thus expectorate any residue.

Such techniques as light pressure upward on the thyroid cartilage to assist in laryngeal elevation are of questionable impact.

Reduced Laryngeal Closure. Exercises to improve laryngeal adduction during swallowing have been outlined in the section on indirect procedures for working on swallowing. The supraglottic swallow, or voluntary airway closure, is often sufficient to increase closure in many patients. In this technique the patient is taught to hold his or her breath and swallow simultaneously and to release the air into a cough after the swallow. It is a useful technique because the patient may be directed by the clinician as the individual performs the procedure. The clinician can essentially "cheerlead" as the patient holds his or her breath and continues to hold it while swallowing. A reminder to cough immediately after the swallow is important. It is difficult for patients to remember to hold their breath tightly and to release the air into a cough rather than inhaling first. Obviously, if they inhale first, they will aspirate the material instead of clearing it from their airway. The supraglottic sequence is a technique that can be practiced using "dry swallows" without giving the patient any actual food or liquid to swallow. When the clinician is satisfied that the patient has mastered the sequence, food or liquid can be given. The patient with reduced laryngeal closure may do best with a thicker consistency. However, if the reduced laryngeal closure is combined with a reduction in pharyngeal peristalsis, thinner material will be easier because thicker consistencies will have a greater tendency to remain in the pharynx after the swallow and be aspirated at that time.

Some patients benefit from a forward head posture during swallowing, which again widens the vallecular space. The hemilaryngectomee who has swallowing disorders because of slightly reduced adduction may exhibit normal swallowing without aspiration with the head tilted forward. However, the patient must have an epiglottis for this procedure to be successful. Therefore, it will not work for a supraglottic laryngectomee whose epiglottis has been included in the resection.

Occasionally, turning the patient's head to the nonfunctional side or placing pressure on the thyroid cartilage on the nonfunctional side may improve closure (Buckley et al., 1976). But placement of downward pressure on the head or manipulation of the larynx from side to side or up and down will have little effect on laryngeal closure, and may, in fact, inhibit laryngeal elevation and closure during the swallow.

Disorders Affecting the Esophageal Phase of the Swallow

Disorders affecting the esophageal phase of deglutition are normally handled medically. They may be diagnosed in the radiographic study completed by the swallowing therapist and the radiologist, but will not normally be treated by the swallowing therapist.

Summary

A number of techniques have been discussed here that may improve various aspects of swallowing. They are not intended to provide a cookbook approach to the problem, nor are they presented as an all-inclusive list of management techniques. Often techniques must be combined for patients with a multiplicity of disorders affecting swallowing. It is rare to find a patient with a pure disorder. The most important aspect of management is the accurate diagnosis of the neuromotor or anatomic problem or problems affecting deglutition. Once the specific problem has been defined, the swallowing therapist can design an appropriate program to manage the problem both in terms of nutrition and of rehabilitation of swallowing patterns.

Swallowing problems typical of various patient populations are discussed in the following three chapters.

Establishing the Multidisciplinary Management Procedures for Dsyphagia

As in many other rehabilitation programs, dysphagia rehabilitation is usually best accomplished with a team of professionals, including the radiologist, the patient's managing physician, the swallowing therapist, the nurse, and the dietitian (Larsen, 1973; Newman, Dodaro, & Welch, 1980; Strandberg, 1982).

The Radiographic Procedure

As discussed earlier, the radiographic assessment (videofluoroscopy) of deglutition is of major importance in management. To initiate this procedure the professional designated as the swallowing therapist should be knowledgeable in the radiographic symptoms of the various anatomic and physiologic disorders of deglutition. This individual or the chief of his or her department should meet with the chief of radiology in the hospital to discuss establishing the new X-ray procedure in which both the swallowing therapist *and* the radiologist participate, writing and signing a single report. The swallowing therapist should be prepared to discuss the necessary radiographic procedure and the ways it differs from the standard barium swallow or upper GI examination (as summarized in Chapter 4).

Once the procedure has been agreed upon, the cost of the procedure should be established. In most institutions there are three fees charged: the room fee for use of the equipment, the radiologist's fee and the swallowing therapist's fee. These fees should be discussed with the administrator of the institution involved, as should the establishment of the new procedure. There are instances in which the professional initiating the request for the new procedure should discuss it *first* with referring physicians or the institution's administration before approaching the other professionals involved.

The Multidisciplinary Management Team

Before the dysphagia management program can begin, all professionals involved must know their roles and be fully prepared to handle patients.

The professional designated as the *swallowing therapist* is the key to the success of the team. This individual participates in the diagnosis of the patient's swallowing disorder (bedside and radiographic) and plans the appropriate therapy strategies, in consultation with the patient's attending physician(s). The swallowing therapist works with the patient on specific exercise programs for deglutition, explaining to the patient the rationales for the various exercises. The swallowing therapist should be the only professional to give the patient instructions on swallowing and should be the only person to change these exercises or instructions as the patient progresses. All instructions should be given in writing, posted in the patient's room, and described in the patient's medical chart.

The swallowing therapist is also responsible for communicating each patient's current status, swallowing instructions, and therapy goals to the other members of the team. This may be done in a chart rounds format, by telephone, or in individual conversations. However it is accomplished, excellent communication between members of the team caring for the patient is the essential element to successful rehabilitation of deglutition, as it is in any multidisciplinary team effort.

The *dietitian's* role is to assure that the proper consistencies, temperatures and food choices are selected for each patient and that adequate nutrition is maintained throughout the dysphagia rehabilitation program. This may involve recommendations regarding maintenance of non-oral feeding options or the use of supplements to increase the caloric content of the foods the patient takes by mouth.

The *patient's physician* plays a key role on the dysphagia team in decision making regarding oral/non-oral feeding procedures and medical management procedures, as well as the overall management of the patient. The physician is also important in the reinforcement of swallowing procedures with the patient. The most devastating experience possible during a patient's swallowing rehabilitation is for each professional who comes in contact with the patient to change the therapy instructions. The physician is usually the most significant influence in the patient's rehabilitation. Thus, the physician's consistent reinforcement of the patient's swallowing instructions is extremely important.

Nursing staff may be the first professionals to identify the patient as having a swallowing problem. Their prompt notification of the attending physician and swallowing therapist is important in the total management of the patient. Because nurses usually spend more total time with the patient than other professionals, they are important reinforcers of the patient's regular and correct practice of swallowing procedures. All members of the nursing staff caring for the dysphagic patient should be familiar with the patient's swallowing therapy instructions and be able to give feedback as to whether or not he or she is doing the exercises correctly. If a nurse identifies a patient having difficulty with a sequence of instructions, the procedures should be reinforced or the swallowing therapist called to see the patient again as quickly as possible. It is *always* inappropriate to change the patient's directions for swallowing therapy without discussing any suggested changes with the swallowing therapist. There is nothing more confusing to a patient than to have instructions changed frequently by a variety of professionals.

Education of
Medical Staff

When the swallowing rehabilitation team is trained and ready to begin diagnosis (bedside and radiographic) of patients with difficulty feeding by mouth, the medical staff of the institution must be notified of the availability of the program. This is usually best done with a small meeting format, often at departmental staff meetings. The Departments of Internal Medicine, Neurology, Otolaryngology, and Rehabilitation Medicine are usually targeted first. In each case, the radiographic procedure should be described, highlighting the safety of the procedure for patients who aspirate and the value of the procedure in accurate diagnosis of the swallowing disorder. It is also often appropriate to review the various therapy procedures for particular swallowing disorders. Team participants should be available for questions. It is most important that all members of the swallowing rehabilitation team be prepared to handle patients at the time any announcement of the program is made, as frequently patient flow will be heavy from the beginning. A careful audit of the institution's patient population to identify the percentage of patients with swallowing disorders requiring management is helpful in estimating the amount of professional time required to establish the program.

Bibliography

Aguilar, N., Olson, M., & Shedd, D.   Rehabilitation of deglutition problems in patients with head and neck cancer. *American Journal of Surgery,* 1979, *138,* 501–507.

American Dietetic Association.   Study guide: Dysphagia: The dietitian's role in patient care. Audio cassette series. 1980.

Buckley, J., Addicks, C., & Maniglia, J.   Feeding patients with dysphagia. *Nursing Forum,* 1976, *15,* 69–85.

Davis, R., Vincent, M., Shapshay, S., & Strong, M.   The anatomy and complications of "T" versus vertical closure of the hypopharynx after laryngectomy. *Laryngoscope,* 1982, *92,* 16–22.

Dobie, R.   Rehabilitation of swallowing disorders. *American Family Physician,* 1978, *17,* 84–95.

Ford, M., Grotz, R., Pomerantz, P., Bruno, R., & Flannery, E.   Dysphagia therapy, *Archives of Physical Medicine and Rehabilitation,* 1974, *55,* 571.

Gaffney, T., & Campbell R.   Feeding techniques for dysphagic patients. *American Journal of Nursing,* 1974, *74,* 2194–2195.

Griffin, K.   Swallowing training for dysphagic patients. *Archives of Physical Medicine and Rehabilitation,* 1974, *55,* 467–470.

Heimlich, H., & O'Connor, T.   Patients relearn swallowing process. *Journal of the American Medical Association,* 1979, *241,* 2355–2360.(a)

Heimlich, H. & O'Connor, T.   Relearning the swallowing process. *Annals of Otology, Rhinology & Laryngology,* 1979, *88,* 794–797.(b)

Jordan, K.   Rehabilitation of the patients with dysphagia. *Ear, Nose and Throat Journal,* 1979, *58,* 86–87.

Kirchner, J.   Pharyngeal and esophageal dysfunction: The diagnosis. *Minnesota Medicine,* 1967, *50,* 921–924.

Larsen, G.   Rehabilitation for dysphagia paralytica. *Journal of Speech and Hearing Disorders,* 1972, *37,* 187–193.

Larsen, G.   Conservative management for incomplete dysphagia paralytica. *Archives of Physical Medicine and Rehabilitation,* 1973, *54,* 180–185.

Leonard, R., & Gillis, R.   Effects of a prosthetic tongue on vowel intelligibility and food management in a patient with total glossectomy. *Journal of Speech and Hearing Disorders,* 1982, *47,* 25–30.

Logemann, J., Sisson, G., & Wheeler, R.   The team approach to rehabilitation of surgically treated oral cancer patients. *Proceedings of the National Forum on Cancer Rehabilitation,* 1980, Williamsburg, VA 222–227.

McConchie, I.   Some difficulties in the treatment of dysphagia in adults. *Australia & New Zealand Journal of Surgery,* 1973, *12,* 362–364.

Mitchell, P.   Buccinator apparatus to improve swallowing. *Physical Therapy,* 1967 , *47,* 1135.

Newman, L., Dodaro, R., & Welch, M.   A comprehensive program for dysphagia rehabilitation. Workshop conducted at Mercy Hospital and Medical Center, Chicago, May 29, 1980.

Schultz, A., Niemtzow, R., Jacobs, S., & Naso, F.   Dysphagia associated with cricopharyngeal dysfunction. *Archives of Physical Medicine and Rehabilitation,* 1979, *60,* 381–386.

Silverman, E., & Elfant, I.   Dysphagia: An evaluation and treatment program for the adult. *The American Journal of Occupational Therapy,* 1979, *33,* 382–392.

Strandberg, T.   Establishment of a swallowing rehabilitation program. Lecture presented at workshop on swallowing rehabilitation. Sarah Bush Lincoln Health Center, Mattoon, IL, Jan. 8, 1982.

Trible, W.   The rehabilitation of deglutition following head and neck surgery. *Laryngoscope,* 1967, *77,* 518–523.

Wheeler, R., Logemann, J., & Rosen, M.   Maxillary reshaping prostheses: Effectiveness in improving speech and swallowing of post-surgical oral cancer patients. *Journal of Prosthetic Dentistry,* 1980, *43,* 313–319.

6

Swallowing Disorders After Treatment for Oral and Oropharyngeal Cancer

Introduction

Malignant tumors of the oral cavity can be managed by one of two primary treatment modalities, surgical resection or radiotherapy, in addition to a combination of the two treatment procedures with adjuvant chemotherapy (U.S. Dept. HEW, 1978). Each type of treatment may affect deglutition. Selection of the treatment modality or combination generally depends on the exact site and extent of the tumor. Smaller tumors are frequently treated with radiotherapy alone or surgery alone. Radiation therapy in the oral cavity may be either by implant into the gross tumor or by external beam methods, or both. In combination, an external dose of 5,000 rads is given in 5 weeks with an implant of 2,000 to 4,000 in 3 to 5 days. External therapy alone is usually given to a dose of 5,000 rads over 6 to 9 weeks. The exposed field usually includes all of the regional lymph nodes.

Larger tumors positioned more posteriorly in the oral cavity are most often treated with combined modalities—that is, surgical resection and radiotherapy. Often, patients with such tumors will also receive chemotherapy as a part of their treatment protocol. At this time, chemotherapy for head and neck cancer patients is an adjuvant experimental treatment designed to attempt to control metastatic disease, rather than a primary treatment designed to eradicate the tumor, itself. Many patients will have tumor shrinkage during or immediately after a course of chemotherapy but this is often of short duration. In the case of larger tumors, when both surgery and radiation are used, radiation therapy is considered the adjuvant treatment, designed to control disease within the region of the tumor, while surgery is the treatment designed to eradicate the tumor itself. When surgery is used to control tumors in the *oral cavity,* the

161

general rule is that the malignant tumor must be resected along with a margin of at least 1½ to 2 cm of normal tissue. Therefore, it is easy to see why very small lesions result in large ablative surgeries. Often these surgeries require removal of more than one structure or parts of more than one structure, such as the mandible, floor of the mouth, and tongue. When only one structure is resected, the surgery is known as a simple resection. When more than one structure or parts of more than one structure are included in the resection, it is known as a composite resection. Usually a composite resection includes some part of the mandible. There is one major rule of cancer surgery: no ablative surgical procedure should be compromised because of the desire to maintain the patient's function. Rehabilitation and reconstruction can not be considered until the cancer is removed with normal margins.

Once the tumor and the required margin of normal tissue have been resected, the surgeon can attend to the problem of reconstruction to maximize functional capacity. In some cases, where sufficient tissue remains or where tissue can be borrowed from another site, options are available to the surgeon in the way the defect can be reconstructed. These options, as discussed later in this chapter, will determine how the patient functions for speech and swallowing after surgery. In other cases, where the resection has been very large and little tissue remains to reconstruct the surgical defect, the surgeon has fewer choices in the way the patient's oral cavity defect can be reconstructed.

Until approximately 4 years ago, radiotherapy (when given in combination with surgery) was given to the patient prior to surgery. A full course of pre-operative radiotherapy typically involves 5 weeks of daily treatments with a total dosage of 5,000 rads. This amount of radiotherapy is considered a curative dose. However, when radiotherapy is given in combination with surgery, this dosage is prescribed with no intent of curing the tumor, but merely sterilizing the area surrounding the tumor and eliminating all random cells in the region. In some cases, pre-operative radiotherapy was given for shorter periods, sometimes for 2 weeks for a total dose of 1,500 rads.

Currently, when radiotherapy is scheduled as an adjunct to surgery, it is usually given postoperatively. This is because radiotherapy tends to devascularize tissue and make healing after surgery difficult. As in pre-operative therapy, the full course lasts for 5 to 6 weeks to a dose of 5,000 to 5,500 rads. When postoperative radiotherapy is used, the patient is operated on and the surgical wound is allowed to heal. Radiotherapy is then initiated approximately 4 to 6 weeks after surgery, assuming that there are no problems with healing. This is considered to be the optimal time to initiate radiotherapy because cells that may have been released during surgery will be weakest.

When the radiotherapy field includes the oral cavity, careful dental evaluations should be done prior to the initiation of treatments. Radiotherapy has devastating effects on salivary flow, causing an increase in the rate of dental disease (caries). If patients enter radiotherapy with poor oral hygiene and rampant dental disease, the caries will rapidly worsen after radiotherapy. In addition, any teeth that are infected should be removed prior to radiotherapy, as any extractions after a full course of radiotherapy can put the patient at risk for osteoradionecrosis of the mandible. This is a condition in which portions of the mandible become infected and gradually break from the main body of the mandible to extrude or protrude through the soft tissue, necessitating removal of the infected portions. This is an extremely difficult condition to manage once it has been initiated and should be avoided at all costs by preventive evaluation before radiotherapy.

Tumor Staging

Tumors in the oral cavity are staged according to size and location (American Joint Committee on Cancer, 1980). Tumor staging is generally conducted by the attending physician and permits comparisons of the results of various treatments across patients with the same tumor. The staging procedure creates a standard for comparison of tumor reaction to treatment. Staging for the oral cavity is divided into eight sites, each staged according to the tumor size, nodal status, and presence or absence of metastasis, otherwise called the T (tumor), N (nodal status), and M (metastasis) system. The tumor size or T is assigned a number from 1 to 4, with 1 being the smallest lesion and 4 the largest lesion. Metastasis to the nodes in the head and neck is noted by recording an N followed by a number representing the number of nodes thought to be involved with the tumor. The location of nodes in the head and neck region is shown on Figure 6-1. The M in the TNM staging refers to the presence of metastasis or seeding of the tumor outside of the region. The M is also followed by a number, indicating the number of distant metastases. An M1 would indicate the patient had one metastasis in an area other than the head and neck, often in the lung or brain. In summary, then, each tumor is staged prior to treatment using the TNM system, with each initial followed by a number. In general, the larger the tumor the more aggressive the treatment, with T3 and T4 lesions more frequently treated by combined therapies (Givens, Johns, and Cantrell, 1981). At this time combined treatment usually includes surgery followed by radiotherapy with chemotherapy also

FIGURE 6-1
*Frontal and lateral view of the head and neck showing the
location of lymph nodes in the head and neck.*

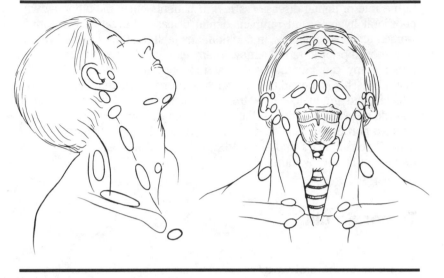

provided, usually initiated pre-operatively and continuing for some time
postoperatively. The nature and schedule of chemotherapy depends on
the particular protocol (study) underway.

Typical Tumor Locations
and Resections in
the Oral Cavity

Tumors in the oral cavity most frequently occur in the six locations
shown on Figure 6-2: the anterior floor of the mouth or the lower alveolar
ridge in the anterior floor of the mouth, the tongue (either anteriorly or
laterally), the lateral floor of the mouth or lateral alveolar ridge, the tonsil
(between the pillars of fauces), the base of tongue area, the hard palate,
and the soft palate. A small tumor located on the anterior floor of the
mouth under the tongue, as shown in Figure 6-3, or on the alveolar ridge
in the anterior floor of the mouth can frequently be treated by a small
resection including only tissues of the floor of the mouth or the rim of the

FIGURE 6-2
Frontal view of the oral cavity showing five typical locations of tumors in the oral cavity and oropharynx.

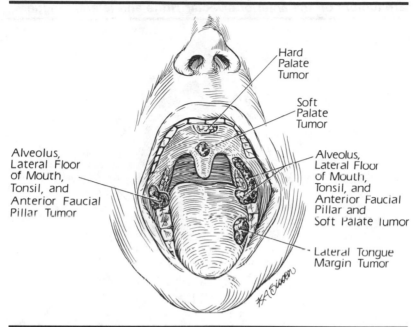

Hard Palate Tumor

Soft Palate Tumor

Alveolus, Lateral Floor of Mouth, Tonsil, and Anterior Faucial Pillar Tumor

Alveolus, Lateral Floor of Mouth, Tonsil, and Anterior Faucial Pillar and Soft Palate Tumor

Lateral Tongue Margin Tumor

mandible as shown in Figure 6-4 (Som & Nussbaum, 1971). Larger tumors in this region often require a composite resection, removal of parts of more than one structure including the floor of the mouth, a portion of the mandible, and often a portion of the tongue, as well as a radical neck dissection on the side of the tumor (Kremen, 1951) as shown in Figure 6-5. This tissue is removed *en bloc* so that tissues which may contain cancerous cells are taken in continuity, and the cancer is not spread by the surgical procedure, itself. Resection of the anterior floor of mouth and anterior mandible frequently results in an "Andy Gump" appearance, i.e. with the mandible smaller and retracted in relation to the maxilla.

Small tumors on the lateral margin or anterior portion of the tongue, as shown in Figure 6-6 often can be removed by resecting only tongue tissue. Larger tumors of the tongue may also be treated with a simple resection of part or all of the tongue (total glossectomy). If the tumors are close to or involve adjacent tissues, such as the alveolar ridge of the mandible or the floor of the mouth, a composite resection may be necessary, including not only the tongue but the alveolar ridge or a larger

FIGURE 6-3
Frontal view of the oral cavity with the tongue elevated so that a tumor of the anterior floor of the mouth is clearly visible as are tumors on the anterior alveolar ridge and lateral tongue.

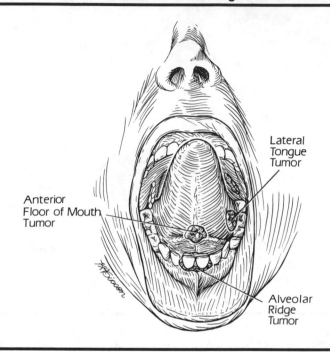

Lateral Tongue Tumor

Anterior Floor of Mouth Tumor

Alveolar Ridge Tumor

portion of the mandible and the floor of the mouth. Often, a radical neck dissection is also included in the resection on the side of the tumor.

A tumor occurring on the lateral floor of the mouth, if small, may be treated with wide local excision including only tissues of the floor of the mouth. However as is more likely, a larger tumor may require removal of not only part of the floor of the mouth, but the portion of the lateral mandible adjacent to the tumor and a part of the tongue, as well as a radical neck dissection on the side of the tumor as shown in Figure 6-7. If the mandible is not invaded by tumor, it may be spared from resection, and simply split vertically, swung out of the way to facilitate the resection, and wired back in place.

A tumor in the tonsil or base of tongue area usually requires a composite resection including removal of the tonsilar area, a portion of the base of the tongue, and a portion of the lateral mandible, with a radical neck dissection (Givens et al., 1981). If the tumor spreads up the faucial arches,

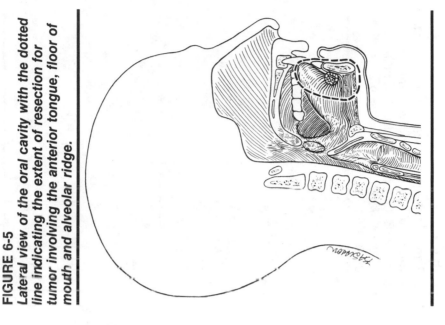

FIGURE 6-5
Lateral view of the oral cavity with the dotted line indicating the extent of resection for tumor involving the anterior tongue, floor of mouth and alveolar ridge.

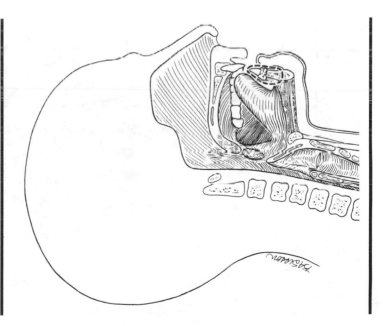

FIGURE 6-4
Lateral view of the oral cavity with the dotted line indicating the extent of resection for tumor involving the anterior alveolar ridge.

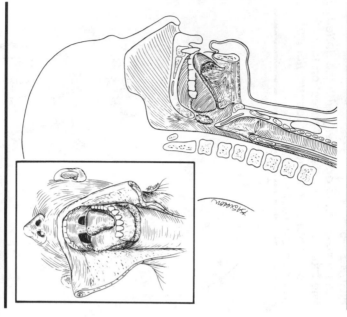

FIGURE 6-7
Lateral and frontal (inset) view of the oral cavity resection for a lateral floor of mouth tumor, including a portion of the lateral mandible, tongue, floor of mouth, and possibly a radical neck dissection.

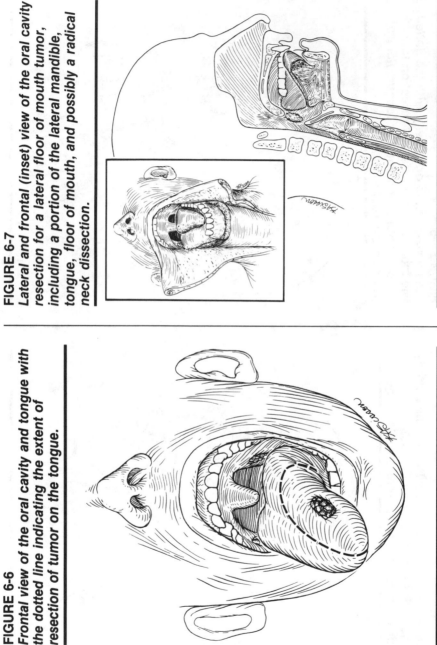

FIGURE 6-6
Frontal view of the oral cavity and tongue with the dotted line indicating the extent of resection of tumor on the tongue.

a portion of the soft palate and pharyngeal wall may also need to be excised.

A small tumor located on the hard palate may require only partial resection of the maxilla. Total removal of the hard palate may be necessary if the tumor is large in size. Tumors on the soft palate may likewise require partial or total removal of the soft palate. In general, rehabilitation of the patient who has had total removal of the soft palate is easier than rehabilitation of the patient with partial removal of the velum. The prosthodontist can more easily develop a prosthesis that adequately occludes the velopharyngeal port when there is no scar tissue present, than when there is a portion of the soft palate which is scarred down and relatively immobile.

Types of Reconstruction
Following the Ablative Procedure

If the resection of tissue is relatively small, the wound may be closed with *primary closure*. That is, the soft tissues remaining are simply pulled together and sutured. Small lesions of the tongue are often closed primarily because the tongue is composed of viable muscle which can be easily closed upon itself, as shown in Figure 6-8. Similarly, if the removal of tissues from the soft palate is small, the remaining tissues may be pulled together and sutured. More often, the resection of tissues is so large that there is not sufficient tissue remaining to permit primary closure. Or, if primary closure were accomplished, the natural tension or pull of the tissue after closure would be sufficient to separate the tissues, create a fistula or reopening of the wound, and prevent healing. Therefore, in order to be able to close the surgical defect, the surgeon may need to borrow tissue from another area of the body. Most often this is done by means of a flap or a graft (Sisson & Goldstein, 1970).

A flap is a piece of tissue which has been elevated or raised away from its normal site. One portion is left attached to its donor site to allow the flap to receive a blood supply from its donor site. The connecting bridge of remaining tissue permits a supply of blood to feed the flap until the portion that is sewn into the wound has an opportunity to heal in place.

Flaps are divided into local and distant types. A local flap is one that uses tissue in an area close to the surgical defect. For example, if a portion of the anterior floor of the mouth is resected along with a portion of the mandible, a tongue flap may be raised to fill the defect. In this instance, a

FIGURE 6-8
Frontal view of the oral cavity and tongue showing primary closure of the tongue after tumor resection.

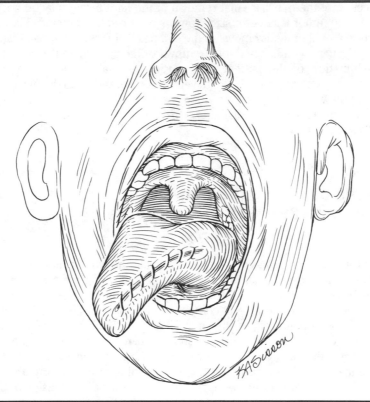

portion of the tongue is sliced horizontally with the posterior attachment to the tongue remaining. The anterior portion of the tongue flap is laid down in the surgical defect, as shown in Figure 6-9 (Som & Nussbaum, 1971). In this procedure, a piece of lingual tissue fills the surgical defect but remains attached to the tongue posteriorly. In many cases, this particular flap does not restrict remaining tongue movement but does reduce to some extent the bulk of the tongue anteriorly. A tongue flap used to close an oral cavity defect would be considered a local flap as it is tissue taken from the immediate region of the surgical defect.

Two other popular flaps are the myocutaneous flap and the skin flap. The skin flap consists of skin and subcutaneous tissue that is moved from one part of the body to another, while a pedicule or attachment is maintained between it and the body for nourishment. Skin may be taken from

FIGURE 6-9
Frontal view of the oral cavity after resection for a lateral floor of mouth tumor. The resection included lateral mandible and lateral floor of mouth which was reconstructed with a tongue flap.

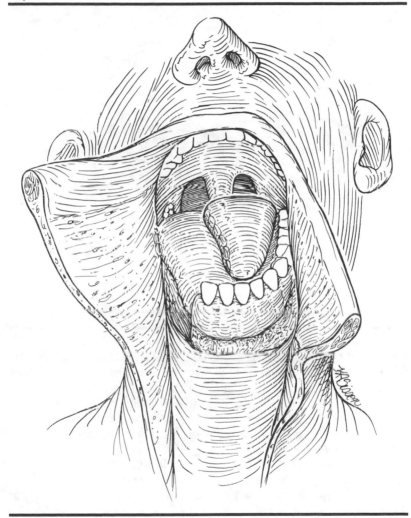

the forehead, neck, shoulder, chestwall, and nasolabial fold, for example, to fill a floor of mouth defect.

When a large amount of tissue is necessary to close a surgical gap, occasionally distant flaps are used. The myocutaneous flap includes

FIGURE 6-10
Closure of an anterior floor of mouth defect with a myocutaneous flap.

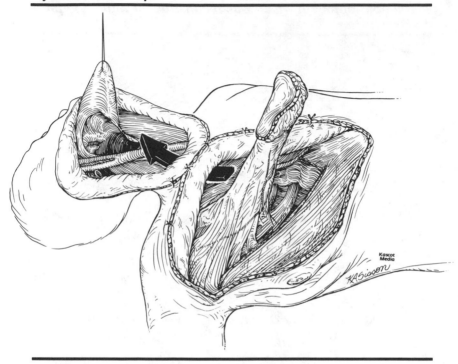

muscle and overlying skin. When added bulk is needed in wound closure, the myocutaneous flap is thought to be more appropriate than a skin flap. The pectoralis major, platysma, and trapizeus are frequently used as myocutaneous flaps in reconstruction of the oral cavity, as shown in Figure 6-10. The myocutaneous flap is usually passed beneath the skin to the reconstruction site, and the donor site is closed at the primary surgery, so that a two stage approach is not necessary.

Microsurgical techniques are being used in relatively few instances to transplant tissue from far distant parts of the body into the oral cavity, with veins and arteries anastomosed or attached carefully to blood supply at the site to assure viability of the tissue. Often called a microvascular free tissue transfer or graft (Zuker, Rosen, Palmer, Sutton, McKee, & Manktelow, 1980), the free flap is a portion of tissue, entirely supplied by a specific artery and drained by a specific vein. It is capable of being revascularized by microvascular techniques at a new site attaching arteries and veins from the recipient site to the tissue transfer. The donor sites for these flaps is less conspicuous than conventional flaps and can be used when conventional flaps may be difficult to use. However, these surgical techniques are time-consuming. Also, infection in the oral cavity after microsurgical procedures, with subsequent loss of the graft, can be a complication. Therefore, these techniques are not yet widely used.

Swallowing Disorders Related to Specific Surgical Resections and Reconstruction Techniques

The two most important pieces of information needed by the swallowing therapist to understand the oral cancer patient's swallowing difficulties are: (1) the exact nature and extent of the resection which was necessary to totally remove the tumor, and (2) the exact nature of the reconstruction of the oral cavity (Logemann, Fisher, & Bytell, 1977; Rappaport, Shrameck, & Brummett, 1967; Rappaport, Swirsky, & Chie, 1968; Trible, 1967). In patients who have had less than 50% of their tongue resected in the surgical procedure, it is the nature of the reconstruction that determines the pattern of function for both speech and swallowing. In patients with greater than 50% of the tongue resected in the procedure, the extent of resection, as well as the nature of reconstruction, determines the functional abilities of the patient. Thus, the first piece of information the swallowing therapist should ask the surgeon before seeing a postsurgical oral cancer patient, is the exact nature of the resection and the reconstruction. It is best for the therapist not to use labels for surgical procedures such as "anterior floor of mouth," or "composite resection," but to ask the surgeon to define, in terms of the structures involved, the exact nature of the surgical resection and the reconstruction. Surgical labels often cover a wide variety of specific resections and reconstructions and are misleading to the therapist.

Partial Tongue Resection

Patients whose surgical resection is small (less than 50%) and limited to the tongue with no other tissues involved, and whose reconstruction is by primary closure (pulling the remaining tissues of the tongue together and suturing) will have swallowing difficulties of a relatively temporary nature

(Conley, 1960). Initially, presumably because of edema, these patients may have short-term difficulties in triggering the swallowing reflex. This may even occur in patients whose resection was not in the area of the tongue adjacent to the faucial arches. Thermal stimulation of the swallowing reflex for several days when the patient begins oral feeding can be very helpful. Also, some of these patients will experience a sense of clumsiness with their tongue in both speech and swallowing. Range of motion tongue exercises and exercises to control the bolus in the oral cavity will usually improve their control and their confidence within the first 3 to 4 weeks postoperatively.

In those patients whose resection has included 50% or more of the tongue, more severe effects on both speech and swallowing can be expected. Obviously, lingual peristalsis and control of material in the mouth will be severely reduced, as the patient will not be able to contact the remaining tongue segment to the palate and thus control the movement of food. Usually, a liquid or thinned paste consistency can be managed by tilting the head backward during swallows and allowing gravity to carry material into the pharynx. Some of these patients will need to learn to voluntarily protect their airway during the swallow as additional defense against aspiration. However, if the resection is limited to the tongue, the pharyngeal and laryngeal aspects of the swallow will be normal and the patient will be able to tolerate a backward tilted head posture without increasing the chances of aspiration. Again, range of tongue motion exercises are necessary to get maximum movement from the remaining tongue remnants. Construction of an intra-oral maxillary reshaping prosthesis will often improve swallowing to the point where patients will be able to manage all food consistencies except those requiring mastication. Even so, some patients using the prosthesis and fork or spoon can manipulate food over to the teeth and do some chewing of softer foods, such as spaghetti or chopped meat.

Anterior Floor of Mouth Resection

After anterior floor of mouth resection, the oral phase of the swallow may be impaired but pharyngeal transit will be normal because the surgical defect does not extend posteriorly (Logemann & Bytell, 1979; Shedd, Kirchner, & Scatliff, 1961). The patient who has the upper margin of the mandible and a portion of the floor of the mouth removed, with closure of the defect effected by using a flap of tissue from a site other than the tongue, will generally have relatively few functional changes in swallowing after surgery. Because the remaining tongue segment is mobile and the

FIGURE 6-11
Frontal view of the oral cavity showing lingual labial closure,
i.e., the tongue sutured to the lower lip.

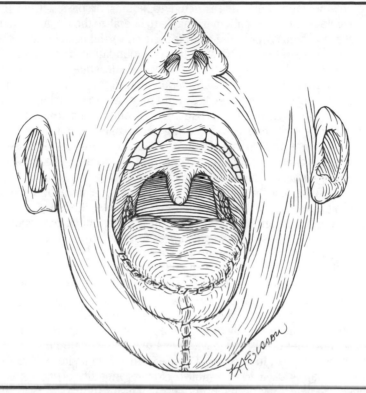

inferior rim of the mandible has been left to maintain its contour, lingual peristalsis is good, and lingual control of the bolus in the oral cavity is essentially normal (Rappaport et al., 1968). There may be an initial period after surgery when swallowing is best accomplished by positioning the food more posteriorly on the tongue. This will speed oral transit time while edema at the surgical site is most severe. Later, the patient will be able to wear a dental prosthesis or full lower denture.

If, however, the same resection of the margin of the mandible and floor of the mouth is closed by suturing the tongue into the surgical defect, as shown in Figure 6-11, the patient will have severe difficulties with lingual control of the bolus, lingual peristalsis, and mastication (Logemann & Bytell, 1979). Because the tongue is sutured down, its anterior range of motion is reduced and the patient's ability to cup and hold material in the anterior mouth in preparation for the swallow is severely affected. Shedd,

Scatliff, & Kirchner (1960) feel that disruption of the mylohyoid support for the tongue contributes significantly to these problems. This can be compensated for by positioning food more posteriorly, but the consistency of the food must be restricted to liquids or pastes. Chewing is impossible because the patient is unable to lateralize the tongue (and thus lateralize the bolus over to the teeth for chewing) and usually cannot wear dentures because there is no alveolus as a foundation. Therefore, unless the tongue is released from this position by subsequent surgery, these patients will be unable to eat any food requiring mastication. If tongue movement is severely reduced, the liquid may have to be syringed into the back of the oral cavity. These patients will often need to be taught to voluntarily protect their airway during the swallow, not because of reduced laryngeal or pharyngeal control in the swallow but because they can lose material over the tongue into the airway before they actually initiate a voluntary swallow.

A composite resection in the area of the anterior floor of the mouth, including a portion of the entire anterior mandible, the anterior floor of the mouth, a portion of the tongue, and a radical neck dissection may result in a variety of swallowing disorders from mild to severe, depending upon the way the surgical defect is reconstructed and the extent of resection of the tongue (Logemann & Bytell, 1980).

Patients who have had the tongue sewn into the surgical defect at the front of the mandible, as described earlier for resection of the rim of the mandible and floor of the mouth, will have severe difficulties in swallowing, similar to those already described because of the severe reduction in tongue movement. This is true whether small or larger amounts of tongue have been resected. In contrast, if tissue from a distant site, a local flap or a tongue flap is used to accomplish closure, mobility of the remaining tongue segment may be good enough to permit functional swallowing. A tongue flap, as described earlier, involves splitting the tongue longitudinally and using one small portion to close the surgical defect while leaving the remaining bulk of tongue to move normally, as shown in Figure 6-9.

Figure 6-12 shows the difference in swallowing transit time based on the method of surgical reconstruction in patients after anterior floor of mouth resection. Three groups of patients were studied at Northwestern, each with only 10% of the tongue resected: (1) five patients who had reconstruction of their surgical defect by tongue flap, as just described; (2) five patients who had their surgical defect reconstructed by lingual labial closure, i.e. sewing the tongue to the lip; and (3) five patients whose closure was accomplished without using any tongue tissue. Those patients with no tongue used in surgical closure functioned most normally, followed by those patients whose reconstruction was completed by tongue flap. Patients whose tongue was sutured into the surgical defect func-

FIGURE 6-12
Oral transit times for three groups of patients with different surgical closure after anterior floor of mouth resection.

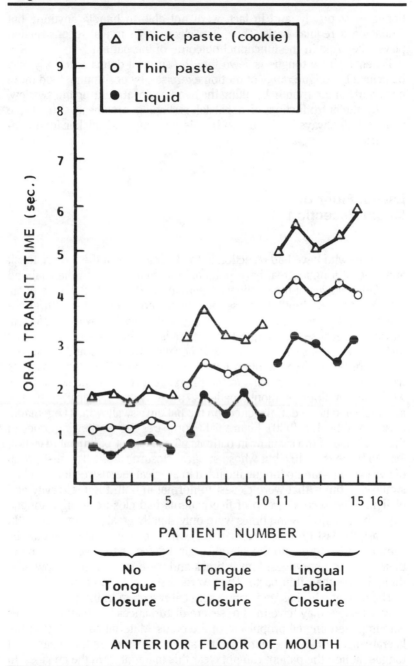

tioned most poorly, and in fact, were not able to handle anything but liquids on a regular basis. Thus, it is clear, that surgical reconstruction plays a key role in the functional outcome of the patient.

Patients whose tongue is sewn into the surgical defect anteriorly may be helped by tongue range of motion exercises, by positioning food more posteriorly in the mouth, by tilting the head backward during the swallow, and by the introduction of a palatal reshaping prosthesis. But, these patients will always be unable to handle chewing and thicker food consistencies.

Lateral Floor of Mouth Resection

Patients who have had resection in the lateral floor of the mouth, tonsil and base of tongue area, have potential difficulties in both the oral and pharyngeal stages of the swallow (Logemann & Bytell, 1979; Shedd et al., 1961; Shedd et al., 1960). Because the tongue and other oral structures are involved in the resection, the oral stage of the swallow will be affected. However, because the surgical resection is in the area of the faucial arches where the swallowing reflex is normally triggered, and because a portion of the pharynx is often involved in the resection, these patients will often also have problems in the pharyngeal stage of the swallow. As with anterior floor of mouth patients, the way the surgical closure is accomplished has a definite effect on the patient's swallowing (Logemann, Sisson, & Wheeler, 1980). Figure 6-13 compares the swallowing times in the oral stage of the swallow in patients whose extent of lingual resection was no more than 10% but whose surgical closure varied. The first group of five patients had no tongue included in surgical reconstruction and had swallowing times that were closest to normal in both the oral cavity and pharynx. The second group of five patients had closure using a tongue flap and their swallowing times were only slightly greater than normal. In contrast, the last group of five patients, whose closure was completed by suturing the tongue into the lateral surgical defect, had severe slowing of their oral and pharyngeal transit times and were unable to swallow anything thicker than thin paste. They were also unable to chew.

The patient who has undergone surgical resection in the tonsil/base of tongue region, may have mild to severe disturbances in oral transit times with impaired lingual propulsion of the bolus. Material can collect in the lateral sulcus or on the hard palate, and because of reduced range of tongue motion the patient can not clear this material from the crevices. In

FIGURE 6-13
Oral transit times for three groups of patients with different surgical closure after lateral floor of mouth resection.

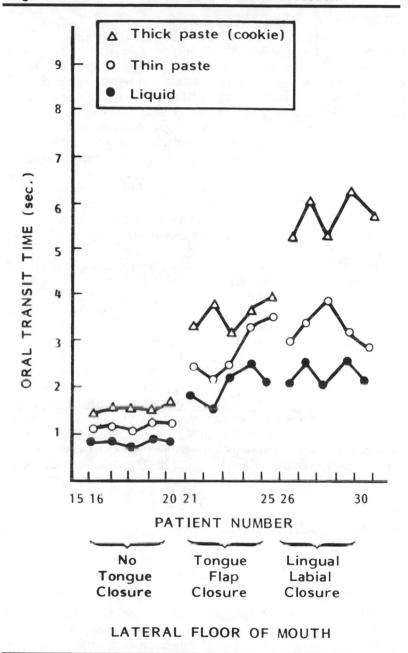

addition to these oral problems, the surgical resection is located in the area of the faucial arches where the swallowing reflex is triggered. Thus, these patients may have delayed or reduced triggering of the swallowing reflex. When the reflex does trigger, patients may have reduced pharyngeal peristalsis causing a residue of material to remain in the pharynx after the swallow. Usually their laryngeal control in swallowing is normal unless a fistula has developed in healing, causing scar tissue to form in the pharynx that can inhibit laryngeal elevation. A fistula in the pharynx causing scar tissue can also lead to a slight defect, or crevice, that collects material. Therapy to improve tongue range of motion, improve triggering of the swallowing reflex, and promote voluntary protection of the airway during the swallow and clearing of the pharynx after the swallow are often helpful. Occasionally following this type of resection, these patients have difficulty with the cricopharyngeal sphincter so that it does not open appropriately during swallowing. A cricopharyngeal myotomy in these cases may be appropriate.

These patients often benefit from a maxillary reshaping prosthesis. If the patient has teeth, the maxillary prosthesis can be made to clip onto the teeth. If the patient is edentulous, the maxillary prosthesis can be retained by suction. In edentulous patients whose resection included part of the mandible, the purpose of the prosthesis is to speed oral and pharyngeal transit times and to facilitate chewing, if possible. However, many patients with composite resection of the lateral floor of the mouth, tongue, and mandible who have no teeth and whose closure has been accomplished by suturing the tongue into the deficit, cannot have a lower denture made to fit their altered anatomy postoperatively. Even those patients who have a more mobile tongue and who have mandibular reconstruction at some time after their original ablative surgical procedure will usually not enjoy significant functional improvement or be able to wear a lower denture (Lawson, Balk, Loscalzo, Biller, & Krespi, 1982; Rappaport et al., 1968).

Swallowing Disorders after Radiotherapy to the Oral Cavity

During a full course of radiotherapy to the oral cavity patients often experience reduced saliva flow, edema, and occasionally, sores in the mouth. Patients with dentures or prostheses may need to discontinue wearing these during and immediately after radiotherapy, as the contact of the denture or prosthesis against the oral tissues may create irritation and open sores that will have difficulty healing because of the radiotherapy. Prior to and during radiotherapy to the oral cavity, each patient should have regular fluoride treatment to prevent caries (Fleming, 1982). Some patients experience a diminishing of the swallowing reflex during or sometimes after radiotherapy. Other than possible reduced saliva flow, tenderness, and swelling, this reduced swallowing reflex is the most frequent sequela to radiation therapy of the oral cavity. Not all radiotherapy effects occur during or immediately after the series of treatments. Occasionally, irradiated patients will develop swallowing problems a year or two after the completion of radiotherapy, and fluoroscopic examination most frequently reveals a delayed swallowing reflex and reduced pharyngeal peristalsis.

General Principles of Swallowing Therapy with Treated Oral Cancer Patients

It is important to talk with the patients pre-operatively to discuss potential swallowing problems. It is impossible to know the exact extent of the swallowing disorder that will occur postoperatively, but it is important to alert the patient that problems may be encountered with swallowing after the surgery and to provide reassurance that the swallowing therapist will be available to provide any necessary exercise programs. The patient must be informed that he or she has some responsibility for his or her own rehabilitation by cooperating with and carrying through exercise programs. It is most difficult to initiate treatment postoperatively with a patient who has been unprepared for any problems with swallowing. Many patients will assume that their swallowing will recover normally without any effort on their part. When it becomes clear after several weeks in the hospital that swallowing will not improve spontaneously, patients can become quite depressed. Thus, pre-operative discussions of the potential need for therapy to improve swallowing can reduce the patient's emotional reaction to unanticipated problems.

Swallowing therapy, including those preparatory oromotor exercises that are necessary to build muscle control for swallowing, are begun when the surgeon indicates that the patient's healing has progressed to the point where there is no danger to suture lines. In patients without complications, this is usually within 10 to 14 days after surgery. At that time, an aggressive program of tongue range of motion exercises and jaw range of motion exercises is begun. Jaw range of motion exercises are particularly important if the patient will undergo post-operative radiotherapy and should be continued throughout radiotherapy and for 4 to 6 weeks after the completion of the radiation treatments. Radiotherapy will cause an increase in fibrosis in the muscles of mastication which will reduce mandibular opening, sometimes to within 1 cm. Fibrosis makes future dental work and the development of any prosthetic appliances difficult. It is easier to ameliorate this condition if the patient continues active jaw range of motion exercises through and after radiotherapy, rather than beginning the exercises after the condition has occurred, at 1 to 2 months after the completion of radiotherapy (Fleming, 1982).

Swallowing therapy is usually begun when the patient is still in the hospital and has a nasogastric tube in place to maintain nutrition. After the complete assessment of oral functioning and initiation of range of motion exercises, a videofluoroscopic examination of swallowing is completed using the three materials, liquid, paste, and cookie. The therapy program is then designed to improve any dysfunctions noted on the fluoroscopy. Most often, patients can begin oral feeding at that time with some consistency of food, usually liquid. As oral function improves, the consistency of the material can be gradually increased.

Therapy then continues until a patient's swallowing has reached a point where the therapist and the patient agree that maximum goals have been attained. This usually involves following the patient weekly for 2 to 3 months on an outpatient basis, and may include developing a prosthesis with a maxillofacial prosthodontist, as well as working on more difficult tongue exercises to improve control of the bolus (Logemann, 1983; Logemann et al., 1980; Wheeler, Logemann, & Rosen, 1980). Some patients, for example those who have undergone a composite resection including an extensive tongue resection (75% or more) and a partial mandibulectomy, will never be able to chew—so their diet will always be restricted to liquids and soft foods. Often, the ultimate functional outcome cannot be determined until several months postoperatively, and then involves discussions between the various members of the team seeing the patient.

Normally, maximum rehabilitation goals in head and neck cancer patients can only be attained with a team of professionals seeing the patient, including nursing staff, speech pathologist/swallowing therapist, social worker, dentist, and maxillofacial prosthodontist. It is usually the social worker, speech pathologist, and maxillofacial prosthodontist who follow the patient most intensively after hospital discharge, and work to define maximum obtainable functional goals. It is often not possible to know the patient's capabilities until the speech pathologist and maxillofacial prosthodontist have had an opportunity to work together to develop optimum prosthetic interventions to assist the patient in his or her rehabilitation.

Bibliography

American Joint Committee on Cancer. *Staging of cancer head and neck sites.* Chicago: Author, 1980.

Aguilar, N., Olson, M., & Shedd, D. Rehabilitation of deglutition problems in patients with head and neck cancer. *American Journal of Surgery,* 1979, *138,* 501–507.

Asamoah, D. Pseudotumors of the oropharynx due to muscular contraction. *Clinical Radiology,* 1979, *30,* 485–488.

Baek, S., Biller, H., Krespi, Y., & Lawson, W. The pectoralis major myocutaneous island flap for reconstruction of the head and neck. *Head and Neck Surgery,* 1979, *1,* 293–300.

Brewin, T. Alcohol shift and alcohol dysphagia in Hodgkins disease carcinoma of cervix and other neoplasms. *British Journal of Cancer,* 1966, *20,* 688–702.

Conley, J. Swallowing dysfunctions associated with radical surgery of the head and neck. *Archives of Surgery,* 1960, *80,* 602–612.

Dingman, D. Postoperative management of the severe oral cripple. *Plastic and Reconstructive Surgery,* 1970, *45,* 263–267.

Doberneck, R., & Antoine, J. Deglutition after resection of oral, laryngeal, and pharyngeal cancers. *Surgery,* 1974, *75,* 87–90.

Downie, P. The rehabilitation for patients following head and neck surgery. *Journal of Laryngology and Otology,* 1975, *89,* 1281–1284.

Fleming, I. Dental care for cancer patients receiving radiotherapy to the head and neck. *The Cancer Bulletin,* 1982, *34,* 63–65.

Givens, C., Johns, M., & Cantrell, R. Carcinoma of the tonsil. *Archives of Otolaryngology,* 1981, *107,* 730–734.

Gluckman, J., McDonough, J., Donegan, J., Crissman, J., Fullen, W., & Shumrick, D. The free jejunal graft in head and neck reconstruction. *Laryngoscope,* 1981, *91,* 1887–1895.

Grabb, W., & Myers, M. (Eds.). *Skin flaps.* Boston: Little, Brown & Co., 1975.

Jabaley, M., & Hoopes, J. A simple technic for laryngeal suspension after partial or complete resection of the hyomandibular complex. *American Journal of Surgery,* 1969, *118,* 685–690.

Kremen, A. Cancer of the tongue. A surgical technique for a primary combined enbloc resection of tongue, floor of mouth and cervical lymphatics. *Surgery,* 1951, *30,* 227–238.

Lawson, W., Balk, S., Loscalzo, L., Biller, H., & Krespi, Y. *Experience* with immediate and delayed mandibular reconstruction. *Laryngoscope,* 1982, *92,* 5–10.

Logemann, J. Articulation management of the oral pharyngeal impaired patient. In W. H. Perkins (Ed.), *Current therapy for communication disorders.* New York: Thieme and Stratton, 1983.

Logemann, J., & Bytell, D. Articulation patterns of five groups of head and neck surgical patients. Paper presented at the annual convention of the American Speech and Hearing Association, San Francisco, November, 1978.

Logemann, J., & Bytell, D. Swallowing disorders in three types of head and neck surgical patients. *Cancer,* 1979, *44,* 1075–1105.

Logemann, J., Fisher, H., & Bytell, D. Functional effects of reconstruction in partially glossectomized patients. Paper presented at the annual convention of the American Speech and Hearing Association, Chicago, November, 1977.

Logemann, J., Sisson, G., & Wheeler, R. The team approach to rehabilitation of surgically treated oral cancer patients. *Proceedings of the National Forum on Cancer Rehabilitation,* 1980, Williamsburg, VA, 222–227.

Massengill, R., Maxwell, S., & Pickrell, K. A swallowing characteristic noted in a glossectomy patient. *Plastic and Reconstructive Surgery,* 1970, *45,* 89–91.

Mathes, S., & Nahai, F. (Eds.). *Clinical applications for muscle and musculo cutaneous flaps.* St. Louis: C. V. Mosby Co., 1982.

McConnell, F., & Teichgraeber, R. Comparison of three methods of oral reconstruction: Their effects on speech and tongue motion. A paper presented at the American Academy of Facial Plastic and Reconstructive Surgery, Palm Beach, May 1982.

Munson, T., & Russell, N. Status of mandibular implants. *The Cancer Bulletin,* 1982, *34,* 56–59.

Rappaport, I., Shramek, J., & Brummet, S. Functional aspects of cancer of the base of the tongue. *American Journal of Surgery,* 1967, *114,* 489–492.

Rappaport, I., Swirsky, A., & Chie, S. Functional considerations after resection of the hyomandibular complex. *American Journal of Surgery,* 1968, *116,* 581–584.

Shedd, D., Kirchner, J., & Scatliff, J. Oral and pharyngeal components of deglutition. *Archives of Surgery,* 1961, *82,* 373–380.

Shedd, D., Scatliff, J., & Kirchner, J. A cineradiographic study of postresectional alterations in oropharyngeal physiology. *Surgery, Gynecology and Obstetrics,* 1960, *110,* 69–89.

Sisson, G., & Goldstein, J.   Flaps and grafts in head and neck surgery. *Archives of Otolaryngology*, 1970, *92*, 599–610.

Som, M., & Nussbaum, M.   Marginal resection of the mandible with reconstruction by tongue flap for carcinoma of the floor of the mouth. *American Journal of Surgery*, 1971, *121*, 679–683.

Trible, W.   The rehabilitation of deglutition following head and neck surgery. *Laryngoscope*, 1967, *77*, 518–523.

U.S. Department of Health, Education, and Welfare.   *Management guidelines for head and neck cancer*, Washington DC: Author, 1979.

Wheeler, R., Logemann, J., & Rosen, M.   Maxillary reshaping prosthesis: Effectiveness in improving speech and swallowing of post-surgical oral cancer patients. *Journal of Prosthetic Dentistry*, 1980, *43*, 313–319.

Zuker, R., Rosen, I., Palmer, J., Sutton, F., McKee, N., & Manktelow, R.   Microvascular free flaps in head and neck reconstruction. *The Canadian Journal of Surgery*, 1980, *23*, 157–162.

7

Swallowing Disorders After Treatment for Laryngeal Cancer

Principles of
Tumor Management
in the Larynx

Tumors in the larynx may be managed primarily by radiotherapy or surgery, with chemotherapy as an adjuvant treatment. For smaller tumors, particularly on the true vocal cord, radiotherapy is the more frequent treatment choice. Cure rates for these small tumors are usually equal with radiotherapy or surgery, with radiotherapy considered the less ablative treatment. As tumor size increases, surgery becomes the treatment of choice. Combined treatment—that is radiotherapy, surgery and chemotherapy—is used in larger tumors, (Goepfert, Lindberg, & Jesse, 1981; U.S. Dept. HEW, 1979).

Tumors in the larynx are also staged, as in the oral cavity, following the TNM classification system. For the purposes of staging, the larynx is divided into three areas: the supraglottis, the glottis, and the subglottis, as shown in Figure 7-1. Approximately 60% of malignant laryngeal tumors occur at the glottic level, 35% occur in the supraglottic area, and 5% are subglottic tumors. In staging of laryngeal tumors the T, followed by a number (1 to 4), represents the size of the tumor, T1 being the smallest tumor and T4 the largest. There are specific definitions of tumor size for each of the three areas of the larynx. The N, followed by a number, indicates the status of disease in the nodes of the head and neck, with the number following the N indicating the number of nodes involved with tumor. An N_0 indicates that no nodes are involved with tumor. As in oral cancer, the M stands for metastasis at distant sites, such as lung or liver. The M, followed by a number 1, indicates one metastatic site outside of the

189

FIGURE 7-1
Lateral and frontal views of the larynx, showing the supraglottic, glottic, and subglottic divisions of the larynx.

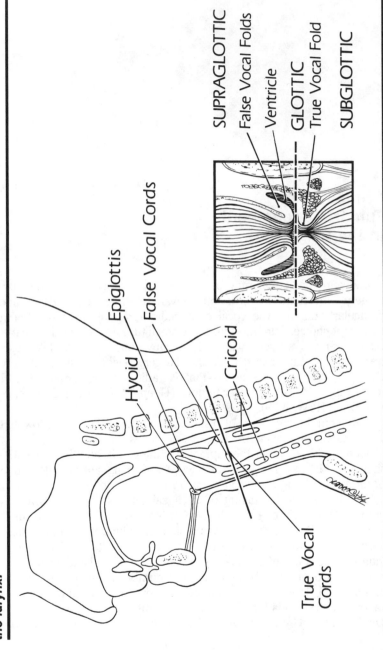

SUPRAGLOTTIC
False Vocal Folds
Ventricle
GLOTTIC
True Vocal Fold
SUBGLOTTIC

Epiglottis
False Vocal Cords
Hyoid
Cricoid
True Vocal Cords

FIGURE 7-2
Superior view of the larynx.

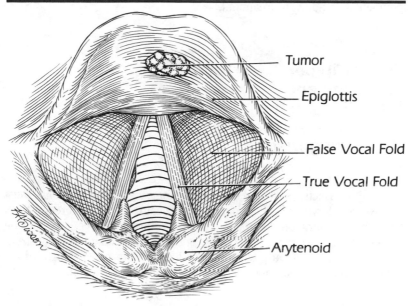

region. Thus, a $T_1N_0M_0$ lesion is a small lesion with no nodal or distant metastasis. The primary physician diagnosing the patient, usually an otolaryngologist or general surgeon, will stage the patient's tumor before treatment, so the results of treatment can be compared with results of other treatments on patients presenting with the same site and stage of disease.

In the larynx, the extent of normal tissue resected along with the tumor depends on the site of the malignancy. Much is known about the lymphatic drainage system and the pattern of spread of tumors in the larynx (U.S. Dept. HEW, 1979). For example, because of the way in which the lymph system drains in the supraglottic larynx, a tumor of the supraglottic larynx (Figure 7-2) will not spread downward to the true vocal cord and/or subglottic larynx unless the tumor is located at the base of the epiglottis. Thus, a lesion on the supraglottic larynx can be removed with a minimum of normal tissue at the inferior edge because tumor cells are known not to spread in that direction. In the larynx, the rule of a 1½-2 cm normal margin is not always followed because of the knowledge of the lymphatic system in the larynx. However, at the superior end of a laryngeal resection, a 2 cm margin of normal tissue must be maintained.

Larger tumors in the larynx are usually treated with surgery followed by radiation therapy. Chemotherapy is often begun pre-operatively as experimental or adjuvant treatment.

Typical Tumor Locations and Resections in the Larynx and Associated Swallowing Disorders

As with resections of the oral cavity, the swallowing therapist must discuss each laryngeal cancer patient's surgical resection and reconstruction with the surgeon. Standard names for surgical procedures can be misleading. Each resection may vary somewhat, as may the reconstruction. The surgeon should be asked to describe the exact structures included in the resection and the details of the reconstruction.

Supraglottic Tumors

Smaller lesions on the supraglottic larynx, predominantly involving the epiglottis (anterior or posterior surface), the aryepiglottic fold or the false vocal folds, are frequently treated with a partial laryngectomy procedure known as a *horizontal or supraglottic laryngectomy* (Ogura, Biller, Calcaterra, & Davis, 1969; Powers, Ogura, & Holtz, 1963; Shumrick & Keith, 1968). A lesion extending below the false vocal cord usually requires a different management procedure. Figure 7-3 illustrates the typical extent of this resection, which generally includes the hyoid bone and epiglottis superiorly, the aryepiglottic folds, and the false vocal folds inferiorly. Even if tumor extends onto the false vocal fold, the supraglottic procedure will take only the upper half of the ventricle, clearly not taking a full 2 cm margin of normal tissue. Again, this is because of the pattern of lymphatic drainage in the larynx and typical tumor spread, which is lateral rather than inferior in a supraglottic tumor. The resection shown in Figure 7-3 might be called a standard supraglottic laryngectomy. This procedure clearly removes the two upper sphincters providing airway protection during swallowing: (1) the epiglottis and the aryepiglottic folds, and (2) the

FIGURE 7-3
Lateral view of the head and neck. The dotted line indicates the extent of resection in supraglottic laryngectomy.

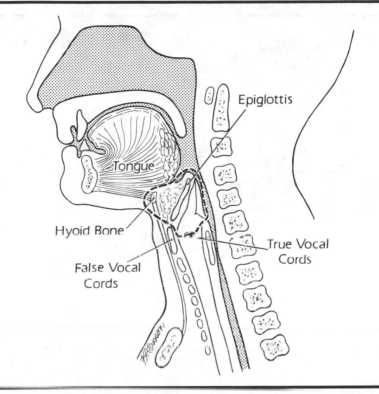

false vocal folds. It leaves the true vocal folds as the only protective mechanism.

In reconstruction, the surgeon usually elevates the remaining larynx and tucks it under the tongue for additional protection during the swallow. Also, a cricopharyngeal myotomy is usually performed during the surgical procedure to facilitate swallowing.

In order to relearn to swallow postoperatively, then, the patient must completely occlude his or her true vocal folds to prevent material from entering the airway during the swallow (Aguilar, Olson, & Shedd, 1979; Sessions, Zill, & Schwartz, 1979; Staple & Ogura, 1966). Laryngeal elevation, another aspect of airway protection, should still be intact. However, because the hyoid bone is removed, laryngeal suspension and elevation are occasionally damaged. After sufficient healing, these patients can be

FIGURE 7-4
Lateral view of the head and neck, with the dotted line
indicating supraglottic resection with extension into the base
of the tongue.

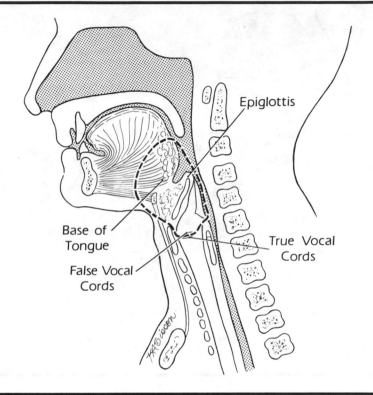

Epiglottis

Base of
Tongue

False Vocal
Cords

True Vocal
Cords

taught the supraglottic swallow, or voluntary airway protection technique. Most do quite well.

The surgical procedure known as supraglottic laryngectomy may be extended either inferiorly or superiorly, depending on the exact location and size of the tumor. If the tumor invades the anterior surface of the epiglottis and extends into the base of the tongue, the supraglottic laryngectomy procedure may be extended up onto and into the base of the tongue as shown in Figure 7-4, the superior limits of resection being at the foramen cecum. Patients who have had the supraglottic laryngectomy extended into the base of the tongue will have a more precipitous drop off from the tongue into the airway. Thus, food or liquid will tend to fall onto the closed true vocal cords, and the closure of the larynx at the level of the true vocal folds must be very strong (Litton & Leonard, 1969; Staple & Ogura, 1966; Weaver & Fleming, 1978). Also, the elevation of the larynx must be intact so the larynx can adequately deflect material (Ogura, Kawasaki, & Takenouchi, 1964). Jabaley and Hoopes (1969) describe a technique for suspending the larynx after resection of the hyomandibular complex. Occasionally, patients with such extended resections may experience reduced lingual movement and control of the bolus so range of motion and bolus control exercises are necessary. Sometimes the sensation in the larynx is reduced because of the sacrifice of one superior laryngeal nerve, with the cough reflex reduced and the patient unaware of any aspiration that does occur. Occasionally too, the swallowing reflex may also be reduced.

As shown in Figure 7-5, the supraglottic laryngectomy can also be extended inferiorly to include part of one vocal cord (Ogura & Mallen, 1965). On occasion, this inferior extension may include part or all of one arytenoid cartilage. Since the true vocal folds and the arytenoids are the only level of airway protection remaining in the patient who has undergone a supraglottic laryngectomy, as this inferior extension includes larger amounts of a vocal fold and the arytenoid cartilage, the patient's chances for recovery of normal swallowing without significant chronic aspiration *during* the swallow are diminished (Lazarus, Logemann, & Jenkins, 1981; Padovan & Oreskovic, 1975). Long-term followup of 25 patients after supraglottic laryngectomy revealed that those patients with a standard supraglottic resection, (that is, a resection that had not been extended into the base of the tongue or the arytenoid cartilages) were able to regain normal swallowing without aspiration *during* the swallow (Lazarus et al., 1981). They were able to swallow a normal diet, including liquids and a full range of solid foods, within 1 month after surgery. However, those patients whose resection was extended to include part or all of the arytenoid cartilage spent a minimum of 2 months and more frequently 6 to 12 months attempting rehabilitation. Several were never able to drink liquids without significant aspiration and always required a tracheostomy tube. Those supraglottic laryngectomy patients who do not have complete vocal fold closure at the time swallowing is evaluated postoperatively, may be put on a program of vocal fold adduction exercises in an attempt to improve muscle function. In general, these exercises will have an effect within the first 2 weeks after initiation. If adequate adduction is not attained after 2 weeks of adduction exercises, a teflon injection into the reconstructed side may be considered—or exercises can be continued, if even slight progress is demonstrated. In managing the swallowing rehabilitation of a supraglottic laryngectomy patient, it is important to assess vocal fold function carefully. Those patients with normal vocal fold function who are able to learn a sequence of instructions will be rehabilitated

FIGURE 7-5
Lateral view of the head and neck, with the dotted line indicating the supraglottic resection with extension inferiorly to include an arytenoid cartilage.

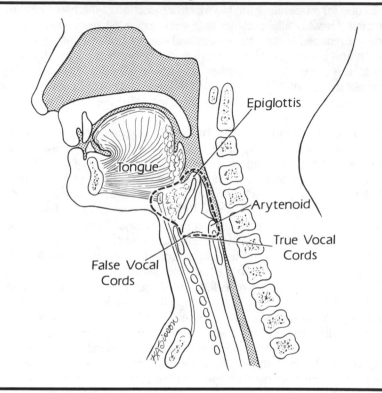

and swallow normally, usually within 1 month postoperatively. One of the criteria for selection of patients to receive a supraglottic laryngectomy is that they must have the capability of relearning a swallowing sequence. Those patients who have mental disorders or who are not able to relearn or follow a sequence of instructions should not be candidates for the supraglottic procedure. If the swallowing therapist questions the patient's ability during the pre-operative counseling and evaluation procedures, the therapist should ask the patient to go through a series of instructions similar to those for a supraglottic swallow and assess the patient's ability to handle them. If a serious question remains regarding the patient's competence after this trial attempt, the swallowing therapist should speak with the surgeon regarding this patient's candidacy for the procedure.

Unilateral
Laryngeal Tumors

Tumors located on the free margin of one vocal fold with only local extension are usually treated with a *vertical laryngectomy* or *hemilaryngectomy,* or *an extended hemilaryngectomy* (Ogura et al., 1969; Padovan & Oreskovic, 1975; Shumrick & Keith, 1968; Som, 1951). The hemilaryngectomy involves physical removal of one vertical half of the larynx, as shown in Figure 7-6, a-c. This resection includes one false vocal fold, one ventricle, and a true vocal fold, excluding the arytenoid cartilage, as well as a portion of the thyroid cartilage on the side of the resection. The hyoid bone and epiglottis are left intact. The patient who has undergone a "typical hemilaryngectomy" should experience few difficulties with swallowing postoperatively because some tissue bulk will be reconstructed on the operated side, against which the unoperated side can attain normal laryngeal closure during swallowing. For normal swallowing, the reconstructed side must be at the same level as the normal vocal fold (Schoenrock, King, Everts, Schneider, Shumrick, 1972; Sessions & Zill, 1979). Occasionally these patients will experience some temporary difficulty with aspiration during the swallow (Jenkins, Logemann, & Lazarus, 1981; Weaver & Fleming, 1978). Usually, tipping the patient's head forward to increase the vallecular space between the base of the tongue and the epiglottis will provide sufficient added airway protection to eliminate all aspiration and allow the patient to resume normal eating. The patient will usually need to use this flexed head posture for only a few weeks postoperatively.

In many instances, the tumor requires that the hemilaryngectomy procedure be extended either anteriorly or posteriorly. The hemilaryngectomy is known as a vertical laryngectomy because one vertical half of the larynx is removed. However, if the lesion is located anteriorly on one vocal fold, as shown in Figure 7-7, the surgical resection will need to include part or all of the anterior commissure of the larynx. In this case, the hemilaryngectomy becomes a frontolateral laryngectomy including approximately one-third of the anterior portion of the larynx on both sides. These patients also are usually reconstructed with some bulk of tissue on the operated side, possibly taken from the strap muscles, so there is something for the normal true and false vocal folds to contact against. The epiglottis and hyoid bone remain, as do most of the strap muscles, for suspension and elevation of the larynx. Both arytenoid cartilages are present so the constricter mechanism at the level of the true vocal fold is intact. Therefore, these patients will probably be rehabilitated quickly also (within 2 weeks postoperatively) (Conley, 1960). However, to

FIGURE 7-6
Three views of the larynx illustrating the tumor location in a standard hemi-laryngectomy (a) and the extent of the surgical resection (b) and (c).

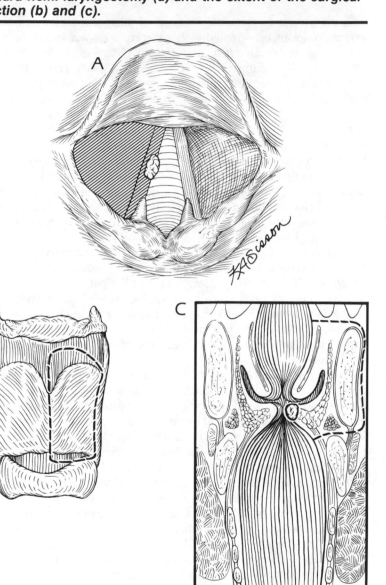

FIGURE 7-7
*Three views of the larynx illustrating the tumor location (a)
and resection (b) and (c) in a hemi-laryngectomy extended to
include the anterior commissure.*

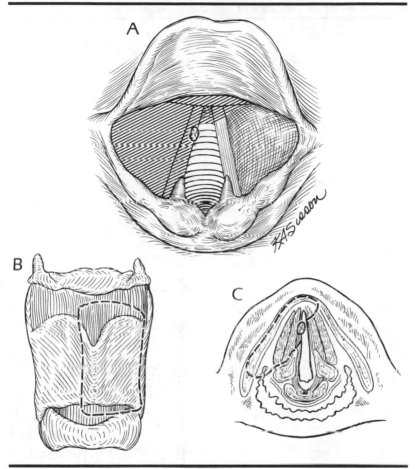

prevent aspiration during the swallow, more of them will initially need the
flexed head posture to prevent aspiration than patients who have undergone the lesser resection.

The hemilaryngectomy may be extended further anteriorly into the
other vocal cord if the lesion is located even more anteriorly. As shown in
Figure 7-8, a-c, the resection can be extended along the anterior commissure to include approximately one-half of the other side of the larynx. This

FIGURE 7-8
*Three views of the larynx illustrating the tumor location (a)
and resection (b) and (c) in a fronto-lateral partial
laryngectomy extended to include the anterior commissure
and the anterior half of the opposite vocal fold.*

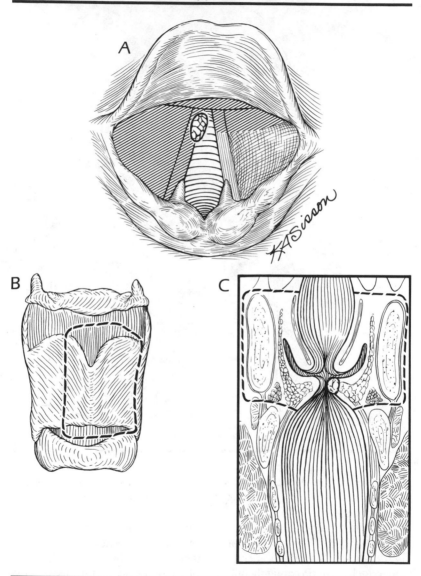

becomes a three-fourths larnygectomy. Because these patients have their arytenoid cartilages intact, a normal epiglottis and hyoid bone, and tissue bulk placed on the operated side to add bulk, there is usually sufficient constriction at the level of the true vocal folds and at the epiglottic level to prevent aspiration. As is true of the extended procedure described previously, even more of these patients will need the flexed head posture in order to regain normal swallowing. Some may also need adduction exercises to improve the sphincteric action for airway protection.

The hemilaryngectomy may also be extended posteriorly to include the arytenoid cartilage if the location of the tumor so dictates, as shown in Figure 7-9a-c. When the arytenoid cartilage is included in the resection, the patient's chances of returning to normal swallowing with no aspiration are greatly decreased (Jenkins, Logemann, & Lazarus, 1981; Sessions & Zill, 1979). A long-term follow-up study of 25 patients who had undergone hemilaryngectomy revealed that those patients with a limited resection resumed normal swallowing within 1 week after initiation of oral feeding postoperatively (Jenkins, et al., 1981). In contrast, those patients who had undergone extended hemilaryngectomy including arytenoid cartilage, experienced a much longer period of rehabilitation. Several of them were never able to drink liquids by mouth because of aspiration *during* the swallow and needed a permanent tracheostomy. Patients with an arytenoid included in the resection will almost certainly require adduction exercises as well as a flexed head posture to facilitate swallowing without aspiration during the swallow.

A number of other partial laryngectomy procedures involving extensive resection of the vocal folds have recently been reported (Pearson, 1981; Pearson, Woods, & Hartman, 1980). Currently, there are no long-term followup studies of the swallowing abilities of these patients. No physiologic descriptions of their swallowing have been recorded other than surgeons' comments that the patients "swallow adequately." Preventing aspiration is a major problem in any extended partial laryngectomy procedure. If aspiration is controlled by reconstructing a narrow glottic chink, the airway is usually compromised and the functional tradeoff for elimination of aspiration is a permanent tracheostomy.

Large Lesions or Those Involving More than One Region of the Larynx

Large lesions (T3 or T4) or lesions involving more than one region of the larynx usually require *total laryngectomy*. Patients who have under-

FIGURE 7-9
Three views of the larynx illustrating the tumor location (a)
and resection (b) and (c) in a hemilaryngectomy extended to
include the arytenoid cartilage posteriorly.

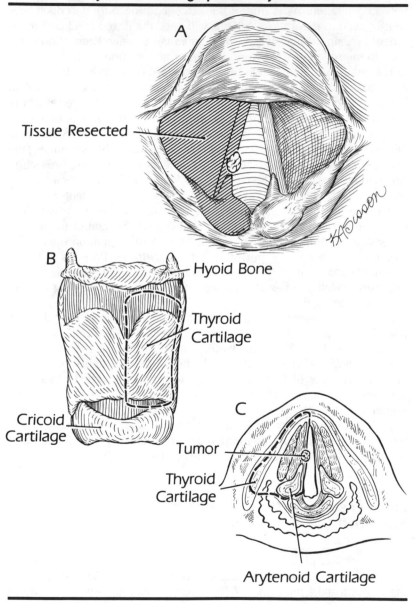

gone total laryngectomy, resulting in a physical separation of the gastrointestinal tract from the respiratory tract, do not run the risk of aspiration of food or liquid. There are, however, several types of swallowing problems reported in total laryngectomy patients. The first appears to relate to the nature of closure of the surgical defect. Some patients will develop a band of scar tissue at the base of the tongue, which was correlated with vertical closure of the surgical defect by Davis, Vincent, Shapshay, & Strong, 1982. These authors hypothesized that the pouch-like recess occurred because the tongue must be stretched in a vertical direction to attain a vertical closure at the base of the tongue. When, in this case, tension is released, the suture folds on itself, possibly leading to the formation of the psuedo epiglottis. The second explanation they propose is that of Kirchner, Scatliff, Dey & Shedd (1963): The suture line at the base of the tongue may break down from tension on the wound edges created by pull of tongue muscles in one direction, and the pharyngeal constrictors in the other. Either of these two hypotheses may be correct. However, other factors in the pharyngeal reconstruction may need to be taken into account. Further research is necessary to define the etiology of this scar tissue band.

On lateral fluoroscopy this scar tissue band appears as a pseudo-epiglottis that forms a pocket at the base of the tongue, collecting food and liquid during swallowing. The effect of this scar tissue band must be examined during deglutition, as it can look deceptively benign when examined at rest. During swallowing, the peristaltic action of the pharyngeal constrictor muscles will pull the scar tissue band posteriorly, widening the gap at the base of the tongue, and forming a large pocket where food can collect. Thus, a structure that looks deceptively small on mirror examination of the base of the tongue at rest, can widen to essentially occlude the pharynx and prevent material from passing when the patient attempts to swallow. Often, the greater the struggle reaction of the patient, the greater the widening of the scar tissue, and the more severe the difficulty in swallowing. Some total laryngectomees are restricted to a liquid food consistency because of this problem. Treatment is generally surgical resection of the scar tissue band.

The second type of swallowing problem which can occur in the total laryngectomee relates to the tightness of the surgical closure. Patients with lesions in the pyriform sinus or extending into the hypopharynx will require more extensive resection of pharyngeal mucosa as a part of their total laryngectomy, thus necessitating a tighter closure. Some patients will form scar tissue strictures in the esophagus after surgery that narrow the esophagus sufficiently to prevent any large amount of material or material of thick consistency from passing through the esophagus. Until recently, the major treatment for this condition has been dilatation. In the dilatation procedure, patients are asked to swallow increasingly larger-sized, mercury-filled rubber catheters which gradually stretch the stricture. However, this treatment has generally been only temporarily successful and has had to be repeated at regular intervals (often monthly). Recently, Singer and Blom (1981) have described a procedure of pharyngoesophageal myotomy after total laryngectomy to release this scar tissue stricture and permit more normal swallowing. According to Singer and Blom (1981), this procedure may also impact on the patient's ability to put air in and out of the esophagus to produce esophageal voice. There are no exercises which will improve such a stricture.

Patients who have undergone total laryngectomy and cervical esophagectomy, whether reconstructed with chest flaps, stomach, or colon, demonstrate no more swallowing problems than other postlaryngectomy patients (Gluckman, McDonough, Donegan, Crissman, Fullen, & Shumrick, 1981; Logemann, 1983). Over the years, a number of surgical and prosthetic voice rehabilitation techniques have been attempted on total laryngectomy patients (Rush, 1981; Shedd & Weinberg, 1980; Woods & Pearson, 1980). In all of these procedures, some method of reconnecting pulmonary airflow to the pharyngoesophagus was attempted. A major problem with most of these techniques has been the aspiration of food into the trachea from the esophagus. One of the most recent of these procedures, the Staffieri neoglottis procedure (Leipzig, Griffiths, & Shea, 1980; Staffieri, 1981), resulted in aspiration in a majority of patients, so the procedure has essentially been discontinued.

The most successful surgical prosthetic procedure, the tracheoesophageal puncture procedure (Singer & Blom, 1980; Blom, Singer, & Hamaker, 1982) involves placement of a small flexible duckbill prosthesis into a puncture wound made at 12 o'clock on the patient's stoma that connects the trachea with the esophagus below the level of the vibratory segment. The small duckbill prothesis placed in the puncture wound prevents the backflow of material from the esophagus into the trachea, so aspiration is eliminated. In addition, the trachealus muscle tends to form a tight seal at the puncture site around the prosthesis, diminishing backflow of material into the trachea from the esophagus around the outside of the prosthesis. Because aspiration is eliminated, the tracheo-esophageal puncture procedure and similar technique, the Panje procedure (Panje, 1981) are the most uniformly successful methods in the long line of procedures that have been attempted to rapidly restore optimum voice to total laryngectomy patients post-operatively. If patients who have undergone any of these procedures aspirate, there is generally no exercise program that will change their aspiration. In the case of the Singer-Blom procedure, the surgeon can cauterize the puncture site to narrow it so the prosthesis better fills the puncture tract.

General Guidelines for Swallowing Therapy with Treated Laryngeal Cancer Patients

Laryngeal cancer patients should be counseled pre-operatively by the speech and swallowing therapist. The therapist should ensure that the patient is aware that there may be postoperative changes in his or her voice and swallowing. The exact nature of these changes is often not known in detail until after surgery, but the patient should be told to anticipate the need for some therapy postoperatively, and helped to realize the importance of his or her participation in any exercise program that may be needed postoperatively. Rehabilitation is much more difficult if the patient is unaware of his or her ultimate responsibility and the need to work actively to rehabilitate his or her swallowing as well as his or her talking.

Postoperatively, the swallowing therapist should review the patient's chart and determine the exact extent of the resection and the nature of the reconstruction. As indicated previously, these two facts will determine the patient's functional capacity after surgery. When the surgeon has indicated that the suture lines will withstand the pressure of speech and swallowing, an exercise program can begin. First, a videofluoroscopic examination of swallowing should be conducted to assess the patient's functioning and define the optimal therapy regimen. Based on this fluoroscopic study, many patients will be able to resume normal eating within the same day if their functioning is found to be normal. If, despite all attempts to increase the force of muscle function, adduction of the vocal folds is incomplete and aspiration is significant *during* the swallow, an exercise program will be necessary before actual oral feeding is begun. Usually, the duration of the adduction exercise program should be no more than 2 weeks before maximum function is attained. However, some patients will slowly improve over many months and be able to resume oral feeding 1 to 2 years after surgery (Staple & Ogura, 1966). Patients should be seen 3 times daily in the hospital and be followed weekly after hospital discharge if necessary. Throughout this therapy regimen it is important for the entire team of professionals seeing the patient to cooperate in the swallowing rehabilitation. It is necessary to continually reinforce the patient's swallowing practice. Consistent support of the nursing service and the physicians involved with the patient is very important. Difficulties arise if 2 or 3 different professionals give the patient different advice about his or her problems. The best swallowing rehabilitation occurs when a single set of instructions are given to the patient and are reinforced by all professionals caring for the patient.

Bibliography

Aguilar, N., Olson, M., & Shedd, D. *American Journal of Surgery,* 1979, *138,* 501–507.

American Joint Committee on Cancer. *Staging of cancer of head and neck sites and of melanoma,* Chicago: Author, 1980.

Biller, H., Krespi, Y., Lawson, W., & Baek, S. A one-stage flap reconstruction following resection for stomal recurrence. *Otolaryngology and Head and Neck Surgery,* 1980, *88,* 357–360.

Blom, E., Singer, M., & Hamaker, R. A tracheostoma valve for post-laryngectomy voice rehabilitation. A paper presented at the American Broncho-esophagological Association annual meeting, Palm Beach, FL, May, 1982.

Calcaterra, T. Laryngeal suspension after supraglottic laryngectomy. *Archives of Otolaryngology,* 1971, *94,* 306–309.

Conley, J. Swallowing dysfunctions associated with radical surgery of the head and neck. *Archives of Surgery,* 1960, *80,* 602–612.

Davis, R., Vincent, M., Shapshay, S., & Strong, M. The anatomy and complications of "T" versus vertical closure of the hypopharynx after laryngectomy. *Laryngoscope,* 1982, *92,* 16–22.

Fu, K., Woodhouse, R., Quivey, J., Phillips, T., & Dedo, H. The significance of laryngeal edema following radiotherapy of carcinoma of the vocal cord. *Cancer,* 1982, *49,* 655–658.

Gluckman, J., McDonough, J., Donegan, J., Crissman, J., Fullen, W., & Shumrick, D. The free jejunal graft in head and neck reconstruction. *Laryngoscope,* 1981, *91,* 1887–1895.

Goepfert, H., Lindberg, R., & Jesse, R. Combined laryngeal conservation surgery and irradiation: Can we expand the indications for conservation therapy? *Otolaryngology Head and Neck Surgery,* 1981, *89,* 974–978.

Jabaley, M., & Hoopes, J. A simple technique for laryngeal suspension after partial or complete resection of the hyomandibular complex. *American Journal of Surgery,* 1969, *118,* 685–690.

Jenkins, P., Logemann, J., & Lazarus, C. Functional changes after hemi-laryngectomy. Paper presented at the American Speech Language Hearing Association annual meeting, Los Angeles, 1981.

Johnson, J., Casper, J., & Lesswing, N.   Toward the total rehabilitation of the alaryngeal patient. *Laryngoscope,* 1979, *89,* 1813–1819.

Kirchner, J., Scatliff, J., Dey, F., & Shedd, D.   The pharynx after laryngectomy. *Laryngoscope,* 1963, *73,* 18–33.

Krajina, A., & Vecerina, S.   Act of swallowing in the fixed larynx. *Acta Otolaryngologica,* 1976, *81,* 323–329.

Lazarus, C., Logemann, J., & Jenkins, P.   Extent of supraglottic laryngectomy and functional status. Paper presented at the American Speech Language Hearing Association annual meeting, Los Angeles, 1981.

Leipzig, B., Griffiths, C., & Shea, J.   Neoglottic reconstruction following total laryngectomy. *Annals of Otolaryngology,* 1980, *89,* 204–208.

Litton, W., & Leonard, J.   Aspiration after partial laryngectomy: Cineradiographic studies. *Laryngoscope,* 1969, *79,* 887–908.

Logemann, J.   Speech therapy after extensive surgery for post-cricoid carcinoma. In Y. Edels (Ed.), *Vocal rehabilitation after laryngectomy.* London: Croom Helm, 1983.

Mann, W., Laniado, K., & Schumann, K.   Pitfalls after laryngectomy and neoglottic formation. *Archives of Oto-Rhino-Laryngology,* 1980, *226,* 207–211.

Ogura, J.   Hyoid muscle flap reconstruction in subtotal supraglottic laryngectomy: A more rapid rehabilitation of deglutition. *Laryngoscope,* 1979, *89,* 1522–1524.

Ogura, J., Biller, H., Calcaterra, T., & Davis. W.   Surgical treatment of carcinoma of the larynx, pharynx, base of tongue and cervical esophagus. *International Surgery,* 1969, *52,* 29–40.

Ogura, J., Kawasaki, M., & Takenouchi, S.   Neurophysiologic observations on the adaptive mechanism of deglutition. *Annals of Otology, Rhinology and Laryngology,* 1964, *73,* 1062–1081.

Ogura, J., & Mallen, R.   Partial laryngectomy for supraglottic and pharyngeal carcinoma. *Transactions of the American Academy of Ophthalmology and Otolaryngology,* 1965, *69,* 832–845.

Padovan, I., & Oreskovic, M.   Functional evaluation after partial resection in patients with carcinoma of the larynx. *Laryngoscope,* 1975, *85,* 626–638.

Panje, W.   Prosthetic vocal rehabilitation following laryngectomy. The voice button. *Annals of Otology, Rhinology and Laryngology,* 1981, *90,* 116–120.

Pearson, B.   Laryngeal microcirculation and pathways of cancer spread. *Laryngoscope,* 1975, *85,* 700–713.

Pearson, B.   Subtotal laryngectomy. *Laryngoscope,* 1981, *91,* 1904–1912.

Pearson, B., Woods, R., & Hartman, D.   Extended hemilaryngectomy for T^3 glottic carcinoma with preservation of speech and swallowing. *Laryngoscope,* 1980, *90,* 1950–1961.

Powers, W., Ogura, J., & Holtz, S.   Contrast examination of the larynx and pharynx. *New York State Journal of Medicine,* 1963, *63,* 1163–1173.

Roed-Peterson, K., Jorgensen, K., & Larsen, B.   The pharyngo-esophageal sphincter after laryngectomy. *Acta Oto-Laryngologica,* 1979, *88,* 310–313.

Rush, B.   New voices for old: Attempts to create a new larynx in the post-laryngectomy patient. *Surgical Rounds,* 1981, *4,* 16–22.

Sandberg, N.   Motility of the pharynx and esophagus after laryngectomy. *Acta Oto-Laryngologica,* 1970, *263,* 124–127.

Schobinger, R.   Spasm of the cricopharyngeal muscle as cause of dysphagia after total laryngectomy. *Archives of Otolaryngology,* 1958, *67* 271–275.

Schoenrock, L., King, A., Everts, E., Schneider, H., & Shumrick, D. Hemilaryngectomy: Deglutition evaluation and rehabilitation. *Transactions of the Academy of Ophthalmology and Otolaryngology,* 1972, *76,* 752–757.

Sessions, D., Zill, R., & Schwartz, J.   Deglutition after conservation surgery for cancer of the larynx and hypopharynx. *Otolaryngology and Head and Neck Surgery,* 1979, *87,* 779–796.

Shedd, D., Scatliff, J., & Kirchner, J.   A cineradiographic study of post-resectional alterations on oropharyngeal physiology. *Surgery, Gynecology and Obstetrics,* 1960, *110,* 69–88.

Shedd, D., & Weinberg, B., (Eds.)   *Surgical and prosthetic approaches to speech rehabilitation.* Boston: G.K. Hall Medical Publishers, 1980.

Shumrick, D., & Keith, R.   Conservation Surgery of the Larynx. Scientific exhibit at the ASHA Annual Meeting, Denver, CO, 1968.

Singer, M., & Blom, E.   An endoscopic technique for restoration of voice after laryngectomy. *Annals of Otology, Rhinology and Laryngology,* 1980, *89,* 529–533.

Singer, M., & Blom, E.   Selective myotomy for voice restoration after total laryngectomy. *Archives of Otolaryngology,* 1981, *107,* 670–673.

Som, M.   Hemilaryngectomy—a modified technique for cordal carcinoma with extension posteriorly. *Archives of Otolaryngology,* 1951, *54,* 524–533.

Staffieri, M.   Phonatory neoglottis surgery. *Ear Nose and Throat Journal,* 1981, *60,* 254–258.

Staple, T. & Ogura, J.   Cineradiography of the swallowing mechanism following supraglottic subtotal laryngectomy. *Radiology,* 1966, *87,* 226–230.

Tomlin, P., Howarth, F., & Robinson, J.   Post-operative atelectasis and laryngeal incompetence. *The Lancet,* 1968, *1,* 1402–1405.

U.S. Department of Health, Education and Welfare. *Management guidelines for head and neck cancer,* Washington, DC: Author, 1979.

Weaver, A., & Fleming, S. Partial laryngectomy: Analysis of associated swallowing disorders. *American Journal of Surgery,* 1978, *136,* 486–489.

Woods, R., & Pearson, B. Alaryngeal speech and development of an internal tracheopharyngeal fistula. *Otolaryngology, Head and Neck Surgery,* 1980, *88,* 64–73.

8

Swallowing Disorders Associated With Neuromuscular Disorders

Two types of neuromuscular disorders affect swallowing: conditions from which the patient can be expected to recover at least in part, such as stroke or head trauma, and conditions that are degenerative in nature, and that will cause gradual deterioration in swallowing ability over time. Management questions for the two groups of patients differ. In the case of patients whose swallowing disorder can be expected to improve, questions to be answered include: Will the patient ever be able to eat a normal diet and if so, when? Is the patient's recovery typical for individuals with this type of lesion? In cases of degenerative disease, the questions include: How long will the patient be able to eat by mouth before gastrostomy or nasogastric tube is necessary? What techniques can prolong oral feeding for these patients? Are there typical changes in swallowing that occur at the onset of the disease and can be used to identify the disease entity? Are there progressive and predictable changes in swallowing physiology characteristic of each lesion location?

Swallowing disorders resulting from neuromuscular disease will be discussed here according to these two types of disorders, those from which recovery can be anticipated, and those that will cause progressive deterioration in function.

Swallowing Disorders Caused by Acquired Neurologic Lesions From Which Recovery Can Be Anticipated

Three types of neurologic conditions may result in swallowing disorders, from which some degree of recovery can be anticipated: stroke, closed head trauma and neurosurgical procedure, and poliomyelitis.

213

Swallowing Problems
After Stroke

Swallowing problems have been reported in patients who have suffered brain stem or anterior cortical strokes (Donner, 1974; Kilman & Goyal, 1976; Meadows, 1973). Typically, patients who have suffered an infarct limited to the posterior cortex with no motor component, will not experience swallowing difficulties unless the posterior lesion creates sufficient edema to affect the anterior cortex.

The swallowing problem most prevalent in brain stem and anterior cortical strokes is the absence or severe delay in triggering of the swallowing reflex. This problem may be present even in patients whose lingual function is relatively unimpaired. If lingual function is relatively normal, the patient will be able to propel material from the mouth into the pharynx using only tongue movement. Material will then fall into the valleculae and rest there unless it dislodges and falls into the open airway. These patients will exhibit much submandibular and hyoid bone movement in their efforts to propel material from the oral cavity with the tongue. These efforts can be highly misleading when evaluating the triggering of the swallowing reflex clinically and can be mistaken for the hyoid and laryngeal movement which occurs as a result of the reflex triggering.

A second problem that occurs less often in stroke patients is dysfunction of the cricopharyngeal muscle juncture at the top of the esophagus (Donner, 1974). This problem occurs in a smaller proportion of stroke patients, perhaps 5%, and is particularly prevalent among those who have had brain stem strokes (Silbiger, Pikielney, & Donner, 1967).

Patients with a lingual hemiparesis may experience reduction in tongue control of the bolus during preparation for the swallow and disturbed lingual propulsion of the bolus during oral transit. If a unilateral pharyngeal paralysis is present, the peristaltic action in the pharynx may be reduced on the affected side, resulting in residue remaining in the pyriform sinus and valleculae on the side of the paresis (Donner, 1974; Kilman & Goyal, 1976). If the larynx is also involved in the hemiparesis, laryngeal airway protection during the swallow may be reduced.

In patients with paralysis of more than one structure in the vocal tract, it is important to initiate therapy to improve: range and precision of tongue movement, adduction of the vocal cords, and stimulation of the swallowing reflex simultaneously. It is often best to work on these motor skills *first* in preparation for swallowing before requiring the patient to incorporate them in a successful swallowing pattern. There is little information available on the pattern of recovery of normal swallowing in patients after cerebrovascular accident. However, data on 75 stroke patients collected at Northwestern University during long-term followup revealed that 62 of the patients who required a nasogastric tube immediately after the incident because of a severely reduced or absent swallowing reflex regained normal swallowing within the first 3 months post ictus. This was in conjunction with active swallowing therapy directed at stimulating the patient's swallowing reflex and other areas of vocal tract functioning. There are no data on recovery patterns without the confounding variable of therapeutic intervention.

If cricopharyngeal dysfunction is the major problem in swallowing and it remains unchanged for the first 3 months post ictus, a cricopharyngeal myotomy may be appropriate. This assumes that spontaneous recovery has taken place and that the residual dysfunction will not change without intervention.

Swallowing Problems Following Closed Head Trauma and Neurosurgical Procedures

Many patients suffer severe swallowing disturbances following closed head trauma or neurosurgical procedures involving the cortex, although the exact frequency of occurrence in these populations has not been assessed. The same two swallowing problems that occur most frequently in the stroke population are also the most prevalent in head trauma and neurosurgical patients: (1) delay in triggering of the swallowing reflex and (2) cricopharyngeal dysfunction. Again, if the disturbance in cricopharyngeal opening is not improved over a 3-month post-trauma period, a cricopharyngeal myotomy should be considered.

Swallowing Problems Resulting from Poliomyelitis

Disturbances in the oral stage of the swallow for poliomyelitis patients may include tongue thrust, reduced lingual control of the bolus, and a disturbed pattern of lingual peristalsis. In addition, many of these patients exhibit reduced pharyngeal peristalsis. Bosma (1953) has described the pharyngeal disorders resulting from poliomyelitis. These include: (1) reduced velopharyngeal closure during swallowing, causing nasal regurgitation, (2) reduced pharyngeal peristalsis, and (3) unilateral pharyngeal paralysis (Kaplan, 1951; Kilman & Goyal, 1976).

Swallowing Disorders Caused by Congenital Neurologic Damage From Which Some Degree of Improvement Can Be Anticipated

Swallowing Problems Associated with Cerebral Palsy

Much has been written about the oral dynsfunctions of cerebral-palsied individuals (Sloan, 1977). The involvement of oral musculature varies widely from one patient to the next. They may exhibit inappropriate reflexive behaviors; an inability to hold material in a bolus, especially if the material is being masticated; as well as disorganized lingual movements that do not contribute to a smooth peristaltic action of the tongue in moving the material posteriorly. Often, as the individual is chewing, particles of food break away and spread throughout the oral cavity. Some of these pieces may fall into the pharynx and from there into the airway. Only rarely does the swallowing reflex trigger when these small amounts fall into the airway, possibly because the voluntary swallow has not been initiated.

There is less information on the occurrence of swallowing disturbances in the pharyngeal and esophageal stages of swallowing in cerebral palsied individuals. In 40 cerebral palsied children assessed at Northwestern University Medical School, the most frequent disorders in the pharyngeal stages of the swallow were delayed triggering of the swallowing reflex and reduced pharyngeal peristalsis. Because of the delayed swallowing reflex that led to the liquid falling into the pharynx and dribbling into the airway before the reflex triggered, these children had difficulty swallowing liquids. The cricopharyngeus dysfunction was rarely a problem in any of these patients. In general, their laryngeal closure was adequate, so that no aspiration was seen during the swallow. Developmental changes in these aspects of swallowing have not been assessed.

Swallowing Problems Associated with Dysautonomia

Familial dysautonomia is an inherited disease with widespread effects including autonomic imbalance, sensory deficits, motor incoordination, and certain episodic phenomena. Some of these children exhibit minimal disturbances with swallowing, possibly some mild reduction in tongue coordination of the bolus, and reduced pharyngeal peristalsis. Other children demonstrate more severe oral involvement and a swallowing reflex that is delayed sufficiently so the children cannot handle liquids (Brunt, Marquiles, Coburn, Donner, & Hendrix, 1967; Gyepes & Linde, 1968; Sparberg, Knudsen, & Frank, 1968). Reduced pharyngeal peristalsis can also be a problem. Occasionally, difficulty with the cricopharyngeus muscle is also observed (Brunt et al., 1967; Kilman & Goyal, 1976; Linde & Westover, 1962; Margulies, Brunt, Donner, & Silbiger, 1968; Pearson, 1979). In addition, manometry has revealed abnormal esophageal motility, an almost total lack of normal peristaltic waves.

Swallowing Problems Associated with Degenerative Neuromuscular Disease

Many of the degenerative neurologic diseases are characterized by swallowing problems that worsen over the course of the disease. There is currently very little information available on the progression of these swallowing disorders, and whether or not the progression is predictable in all patients with similar lesions. Many of the studies that have examined the swallowing problems in neurologic disease have assessed a variety of patients from a number of the disease types rather than looking at a homogeneous group of patients. Other studies have examined a homogeneous disease group but have not categorized patients according to the stage of deterioration in their neurologic systems. There is need for research that follows patients from the onset of their neurologic symptoms to determine the progression of swallowing dysfunction with potential for designing optimum management programs. At present, the armamentarium of treatments for the patient with progressive disease is limited.

Management of the patient with a degenerative neurologic disease often involves progressively restricting the nature of the diet and eventually shifting the patient from oral feeding to gastrostomy. It is important that the patient's swallowing be regularly evaluated so: (1) progressively worsening function can be compensated for as much as possible, (2) the patient is put at minimal risk of serious aspiration and pulmonary problems, and (3) the patient's nutritional status is maintained by initiation of appropriate non-oral feeding methods when needed.

Parkinson's Disease

Patients with Parkinson's disease may exhibit a number of swallowing disorders in all three stages of deglutition (Blonsky, Logemann, Boshes, & Fisher, 1975; Donner & Silbiger, 1966; Hurwitz, Nelson, & Haddad, 1975; Kilman & Goyal, 1976; Logemann, Blonsky, & Boshes, 1975; Nowack, Hatelid, & Sohn, 1977). In the oral phase of the swallow, Parkinson patients exhibit a typical repetitive anterior to posterior rolling pattern in lingual propulsion of the bolus. The bolus is held in a normal position when the swallow is begun. Then the tongue rolls the bolus posteriorly. However, the back tongue often does not lower and the bolus rolls back anteriorly. This backward-forward movement may be repeated a number of times until finally one single anterior to posterior movement of the tongue is sufficient to propel the bolus and the back tongue lowers to allow the bolus to pass (Blonsky et al., 1975; Massengill & Nashold, 1969b). This type of "festination" in the lingual musculature may reflect a form of muscle rigidity—the patient is unable to lower his or her tongue once it has been elevated to hold the bolus in the preparatory position for swallowing.

Some Parkinson patients exhibit a delay in the triggering of the swallowing reflex although it is usually not severe. Once the reflex triggers, pharyngeal peristalsis is often reduced, resulting in residue of material in the valleculae and pyriform sinuses after each swallow (Donner & Silbiger, 1966; Silbiger et al., 1967). This residue typically increases with each consecutive swallow, particularly if material is of a thick paste consistency. Patients in the later stages of the disease may experience sufficient involvement of laryngeal musculature so laryngeal closure during the swallow is incomplete, and some material enters the airway during the swallow. More frequently, aspiration in these patients is caused by the material remaining in the pharynx *after* the swallow falling into the open airway when the patient inhales after the swallow. Occasionally, Parkinson patients exhibit a disorder of the cricopharyngeus juncture into the esophagus. Some authors have reported a higher incidence of cricopharyngeal disorder in these patients (Donner & Silbiger, 1966).

In general, the progression of swallowing dysfunction in the Parkinson patient begins with reduction in pharyngeal peristalsis and the repetitive rocking motion of the tongue. As the disease progresses, the reduction in pharyngeal peristalsis may worsen and laryngeal closure during swallowing may also become inadequate. The swallowing reflex may then become delayed. A cricopharyngeal dysfunction may also occur.

In contrast to Parkinson patients, individuals with essential tremor have been found to exhibit no swallowing disorders (Blonsky et al., 1975).

Amyotrophic Lateral Sclerosis

This progressive disease, involving upper and lower motor neuron damage, often begins with reduction in tongue mobility, so patients become less able to chew and less able to control material in the oral cavity (Dworkin & Hartman, 1979; Kilman & Goyal, 1976). Velar function may become involved so that anterior velar bulging to keep food in the oral cavity during chewing and velar elevation during swallowing are reduced (Robbins, Logemann, & Kirshner, 1982). If laryngeal function severely affected early in the progression, complete vocal fold adduction during the swallow may not be attained and material may be aspirated during the swallow. More likely, earlier in the progression of the disease, pharyngeal peristalsis will be reduced so material remains in the pharynx after the swallow. This material may then be aspirated when the patient inhales after the swallow. Usually at the same time that pharyngeal peristalsis is affected, the swallowing reflex becomes delayed. As long as laryngeal function remains adequate to protect the airway, the patient will be able to feed orally by restricting the diet to liquids and thin paste consistencies.

Twenty ALS patients have been followed at Northwestern University Medical School from the initiation of the oral symptoms until the termination of oral feeding. In all of these patients, the disease began with involvement of oral musculature and later progressed to involve neuromuscular control of respiration and the extremities. The progression of deterioration in neuromuscular control of deglutition observed in 16 of these ALS patients began with reduction in lingual control and pharyngeal peristalsis, followed by a delay in the swallowing reflex. Some patients develop cricopharyngeal disorders, usually as a result of discoordination in the entire pharynx (Smith, Mulder, & Code, 1957). Cricopharyngeal myotomy is far from uniformly successful in these patients, probably because of the severity of pharyngeal, laryngeal, and oral aspects of the swallow, including the timing of the swallowing reflex.

Multiple Sclerosis

Patients with multiple sclerosis have multiple lesions in the neurologic system from the brain stem and cerebellum to the corticospinal tracts. Currently, it is thought that the cerebellum plays essentially no role in the control of swallowing. Therefore, the disorders that these patients have in swallowing relate to their neurologic lesions in the brain stem. Because these lesions may affect single or multiple cranial nerves, the multiple sclerosis patient can exhibit swallowing disorders of various types (Daly, Code, & Andersen, 1962; Kilman & Goyal, 1976). If the hypoglossal nerve is affected, the patient's lingual control of bolus manipulation, chewing, and oral transit will be reduced to some extent. If the Xth cranial nerve is involved, the patient's laryngeal function and airway protection will be reduced. If the IXth cranial nerve is involved, the swallowing reflex may be delayed and pharyngeal peristalsis will be reduced (Silbiger et al., 1967). If all three of these or any other combination of nerves is involved, the patient will exhibit multiple problems. In the 75 MS patients studied at Northwestern University Medical School, reduction in pharyngeal peristalsis and delayed swallowing reflex occurred most frequently in this population. Patients in advanced stages of the disease tended to have a reduction in lingual function and laryngeal adduction as well. However, these latter disorders were far less common and were not seen in all patients with advanced disease.

Myasthenia Gravis

As is well known, myasthenia gravis, a neurologic disease affecting the myoneural junction, presents itself as a fatiguing of the involved musculature with repeated use (Carpenter, McDonald, & Howard, 1979; Donner, 1974; Silbiger et al., 1967). Most frequently, cranial nerves are initially involved and though ocular muscles are most often affected first, any other musculature innervated by cranial nerves may also be involved as the initial sympton (Aronson, 1971, 1980; Carpenter et al., 1979; Donner, 1974; Donner & Silbiger, 1966). Aronson reports a case of laryngeal dysfunction as the first symptom of myasthenia (1974). Two patients have been seen at Northwestern with initial pharyngeal involvement that was only exhibited during deglutition. In these patients, pharyngeal peristalsis was progressively reduced with use until no pharyngeal contraction could be seen. Pharyngeal constrictor involvement as the sole initial symptom of myasthenia is relatively rare, and often difficult to document without fluoroscopy completed at the beginning of the patient's feeding and after approximately 15 to 20 minutes of consecutive swallowing. Patients may be misdiagnosed as having an emotionally based swallowing disorder and referred for psychotherapy or psychotherapeutic treatment. One such patient received 6 months of electroshock therapy for a myasthenic swallowing disorder that was misdiagnosed as a psychiatric disturbance. Thus, it is important for the swallowing therapist to keep myasthenia gravis in mind as a potential etiology for swallowing disturbance, particularly in the presence of a history of difficulty with swallowing which worsens with use and improves with rest.

Muscular Dystrophy

A number of types of muscular dystrophy affect the swallowing mechanism. *Myotonic dystrophy,* characterized by prolonged contraction and difficulty in relaxation of involved muscles, will frequently affect the cricopharyngeal sphincter so it will not relax rapidly during swallowing (Casey & Aminoff, 1971; Donner & Silbiger, 1966; Hughes, Swann, Gleeson, & Lee, 1965; Kilman & Goyal, 1976; Siegel, Hendrix, & Collins, 1966).

These patients exhibit excessive aspiration because the material which cannot pass through the cricopharyngeal juncture overflows the pyriform sinuses and enters the airway.

Oculopharyngeal dystrophy, a muscular dystrophy affecting the ocular and pharyngeal muscles selectively, may result in reduced pharyngeal peristalsis and dysfunction of the cricopharyngeal juncture (Aarli, 1969; Duranceau, Letendre, Clermont, Levesque, & Barbeau, 1978; Kilman & Goyal, 1976). These patients often cannot propel material through the pharynx because of the reduced strength of the pharyngeal constrictors and, in addition, cannot move material through the cricopharyngeus because it does not relax.

Other types of muscular dystrophy may also occasionally affect the pharynx and cause a reduction in strength of the pharyngeal constrictors. This is the most common swallowing dysfunction in patients with muscular dystrophy of any type (Silbiger et al., 1967).

Dystonia

Dystonia is a relatively rare chronic disease characterized by involuntary, irregular chronic contortions of muscles of the head, neck, trunk, and extremities, which may affect speech and swallowing. Bosma, Geoffrey, Thach, Weiffenbach, Kavanagh, & Orr (1982) have completed a detailed study of swallowing in one patient with medication-induced dystonia. According to Bosma, dystonia may worsen with the volitional attempts to manipulate food in preparation for the swallow. As the dystonic movements worsen, the labial seal worsens, and food is lost from the mouth. Collecting the bolus to initiate the swallow is severely impaired, and some material often falls over the base of the tongue prematurely. Oral transit times are slowed, with disorganized lingual propulsion of the bolus. Once the reflexive swallow is initiated, the pharyngeal stage of the swallow is normal with good peristaltic action.

Dermatomyositis

Dermatomyositis is a collagen disease in which polymyositis is one distinguishing characteristic. The polymyositis usually causes dysphagia (Dietz, Logemann, Sahgal, & Schmid, 1980; Metheny, 1978). Reduced pharyngeal peristalsis and dysfunctioning of the cricopharyngeus muscle are the two main problems described in these patients.

Evaluation of the Patient in the Intensive Care Unit

In many instances, the swallowing therapist will be asked to evaluate neurologically impaired patients while they are still in the intensive care unit. Or occasionally, patients will need to be evaluated when they are still comotose. There are several techniques which can be used to assess the patient's swallowing function while putting the patient at minimal risk for aspiration or pulmonary complications. First, the swallowing therapist can evaluate the frequency of swallowing and the apparent strength of the swallowing reflex by resting a hand on the submandibular and laryngeal areas of the neck. This is described in the section on evaluating the reflex at the bedside. Resting the fingers on these structures for a period of 5 or 10 minutes allows the swallowing therapist to assess the frequency of swallowing and the strength of the reflex. Simultaneously, the therapist can assess how the patient handles his or her own secretions. If necessary, the therapist can then open the patient's mouth and attempt thermal stimulation of the reflex using the ice cold laryngeal mirror, size 00. Any muscle contractions in response to the stimulation may be evaluated. After repeated thermal stimulation to the base of the anterior faucial arch, the swallowing therapist may position a very small amount of liquid, generally iced ginger ale, with a straw at the base of the anterior faucial arch and release the material concurrent with the command to swallow. The therapist then assesses the reaction of the mechanism to the presentation of liquid and determines whether or not the swallowing reflex is triggered. If the patient is able to follow directions, a complete bedside examination can be carried out, including assessment of the functional status of each vocal tract structure during volitional and reflexive movement.

On the basis of the results of this examination, the swallowing therapist may ask the patient to repeat several more swallows of small amounts of material as posture is changed so the effect of posture can also be assessed. If the patient is unable to follow directions, the swallowing therapist may be able to perform some informal assessments of vocal tract function and place the patient in particular positions to assess the effects of posture. This full examination involves giving the patient less than ½ teaspoon of liquid and should not increase the patient's risk of pulmonary complications. It is not recommended that the patient be given any larger amount of material until a radiographic examination can confirm the success of the swallowing pattern. Though some clinicians do recommend an aggressive swallowing rehabilitation program to reinitiate oral feeding with very ill or comotose patients in the intensive care unit, the present state of the art in bedside assessment of the functional status of these patients makes the chances for success of such an assessment in this patient population particularly poor and may place the patient at unwarranted risk.

General Considerations in Management of the Neurologic Patient with Swallowing Disorders

In all neurologic patients, sensitivity to aspiration is significantly reduced. Many neurologic patients of all etiologies are unaware of their swallowing disturbances and will deny any swallowing problem. Yet, videofluoroscopy will reveal that the patient is aspirating a significant portion of every bolus swallowed. Apparently, many neurologic conditions affect the sensory feedback regarding position of food in the vocal tract and entry of food into the airway. Whereas many other types of patients are aware of residual material in the pharynx, very few neurologically impaired patients have this awareness. Thus, in assessing and treating the neurologically impaired patient, the swallowing therapist must be constantly aware of the potential for silent aspiration.

Bibliography

Aarli, J.   Oculopharyngeal muscular dystrophy. Acta *Neurologica Scandinavia,* 1969, *45,* 484–492.

Aronson, A.   Early motor unit disease masquerading as psychogenic breathy dysphonia: A clinical case presentation. *Journal of Speech and Hearing Disorders,* 1971, *36,* 116–124.

Aronson, A.   *Clinical voice disorders: An interdisciplinary approach.* New York: Thieme-Stratton, 1980.

Blonsky, E., Logemann, J., Boshes, B., & Fisher, H.   Comparison of speech and swallowing function in patients with tremor disorders and in normal geriatric patients: A cinefluorographic study. *Journal of Gerontology,* 1975, *30,* 299–303.

Bosma, J. Studies of disability of the pharynx resultant from poliomyelitis. *Annals of Otology, Rhinology and Laryngology*, 1953, *64*, 529–547.

Bosma, J., Geoffrey, V., Thach, B., Weiffenbach, J., Kavanagh, J., & Orr, W. A pattern of medication induced persistent bulbar and cervical dystonia. *The International Journal of Orofacial Myology*, 1982, *8*, 5–19.

Brunt, P. W., Margulies, S. I., Coburn, W. M., Donner, N. W., & Hendrix, T. R. The oesophagus in dysautonomia: a manometric and cinefluorographic study. *Journal of the British Society of Gastroenterology*, 167, *8*, 636–637.

Carpenter, R., McDonald, T., & Howard, F. The otolaryngologic presentation of myasthenia gravis. *Laryngoscope*, 1979, *89*, 922–927.

Casey E., & Aminoff, M. Dystrophia myotonica presenting with dysphagia. *British Medical Journal*, 1971, *2*, 443, (Supplement).

Daly, D., Code, C., & Andersen, H. Disturbances of swallowing and esophageal motility in patients with multiple sclerosis. *Neurology*, 1962, *12*, 250–256.

Dietz, F., Logemann, J., Sahgal, V., & Schmid, F. Cricopharyngeal muscle dysfunction in the differential diagnosis of dysphagia in polymyositis. *Arthritis and Rheumatism*, 1980, *23*, 491–495.

Donner, M. Swallowing mechanisms and neuromuscular disorders. *Seminars in Roentgenology*, 1974, *9*, 273–282.

Donner, M., & Silbiger, M. Cinefluorographic analysis of pharyngeal swallowing in neuromuscular disorders. *American Journal of Medical Science*, 1966, *251*, 600–616.

Duranceau, C., Letendre, J., Clermont, R., Levesque, H., & Barbeau, A. Oropharyngeal dysphagia in patients with oculopharyngeal muscular dystrophy. *Canadian Journal of Surgery*, 1978, *21*, 326–329.

Dworkin, J., & Hartman, D. Progressive speech deterioration and dysphagia in amyotrophic lateral sclerosis: Case report. *Archives of Physical Medicine and Rehabilitation*, 1979, *60*, 423–425.

Ekedahl, C., Mansson, I., & Sandberg, N. Swallowing dysfunction in the brain damaged with drooling. *Acta Otolaryngologica*, 1974, *78*, 141–149.

Gelfand, M., & Krone, C. Dysphagia and esophageal ulceration in Crohn's disease. *Gastroenterology*, 1968, *55*, 510–514.

Gyepes, M., & Linde, L. Familial dysautonomia: The mechanism of aspiration. *Radiology*, 1968, *91*, 471–475.

Henderson, R., Boszko, A., & vanNostrand, A. Pharyngoesophageal dysphagia and recurrent laryngeal nerve palsy. *Journal of Thoracic and Cardiovascular Surgery*, 1974, *68*, 507–512.

Hughes, D., Swann, J., Gleeson, J., & Lee, F. Abnormalities in swallowing associated with dystrophia myotonica. *Brain*, 1965, *88*, 1037–1042.

Hurwitz, A., Nelson, J., & Haddad, J. Oropharyngeal dysphagia: Manometric and cine esophagraphic findings. *Digestive Diseases*, 1975, *20*, 313–323.

Hussar, A., & Bragg, D. The effect of chlorpromazine on the swallowing function in chronic schizophrenic patients. *American Journal of Psychiatry*, 1969, *126*, 570–573.

Jennings, G. Uncommon diseases onset with dysphagia. *Practitioner*, 1969, *202*, 808–815.

Kaplan, S. Paralysis of deglutition. A post poly-poliomyelitis complication treated by section of the cricopharyngeus muscle. *Annals of Surgery*, 1951, *133*, 572–573.

Kilman, W., & Goyal, R. Disorders of pharyngeal and upper esophageal sphincter motor function. *Archives of Internal Medicine*, 1976, *136*, 592–601.

Linde, L., & Westover, J. Esophageal and gastric abnormalities in dysautonomia. Pediatrics, 1962, *29*, 303–306.

Logemann, J., Blonsky, E., & Boshes, B. Dysphagia in parkinsonism. *Journal of the American Medical Association*, 1975, *231*, 69–70.

Logemann, J., Fisher, H., Boshes, B., & Blonsky, E. Frequency and co-occurrence of vocal tract dysfunctions in the speech of a large sample of Parkinson patients. *Journal of Speech and Hearing Disorders*, 1978, *43*, 47–57.

Mandelstam, P., Siegel, C., Lieber, A., & Siegel, M. The swallowing disorder in patients with diabetic neuropathy-gastroenterophy. *Gastroenterology*, 1969, *56*, 1–12.

Margulies, S., Brunt, P., Donner, M., & Silbiger, M. Familial dysautonomia. A cineradiographic study of the swallowing mechanism. *Radiology*, 1968, *90*, 107–112.

Massengill, R., & Nashold, B. A swallowing disorder denoted in tardive dyskinesia patients. *Acta Oto-Laryngologica*, 1969, *68*, 457–458. (a)

Massengill, R., & Nashold, B. Cinefluorographic evaluation of swallowing in patients with involuntary movements. *Confinia Neurologica*, 1969, *31*, 269–272. (b)

Meadows, J. Dysphagia in unilateral cerebral lesions. *Journal of Neurology, Neurosurgery and Psychiatry*, 1973, *36*, 853–860.

Metheny, J. Dermatomyositis: A vocal and swallowing disease entity. *Laryngoscope*, 1978, *88*, 147–161.

Nowack, W., Hatelid, J., & Sohn, R. Dysphagia in parkinsonism. *Archives of Neurology*, 1977, *34*, 320.

O'Connor, A., & Ardran, G. Cinefluorography in the diagnosis of pharyngeal palsies. *Journal of Laryngology and Otology*, 1976, *90*, 1015–1019.

Palmer, E.   Dysphagia in parkinsonism. *Journal of the American Medical Association,* 1974, *229,* 1349.

Pearson, J.   Familial dysautonomia (A brief review). *Journal of the Autonomic Nervous System,* 1979, *1,* 119–126.

Richmond, W., Storey, A., & Doty, R.   Integration of deglutition after various transections of medulla oblongata. *Physiologist,* 1960–1961, *3–4,* 94.

Robbins, J., Logemann, J., & Kirshner, H.   Velopharyngeal activity during speech and swallowing in neurologic disease. Paper presented at the American Speech-Language-Hearing Association annual meeting, Toronto, 1982.

Schatzki, R.   Globus hystericus (globus sensation). *New England Journal of Medicine,* 1964, *270,* 676.

Schleider, M., & Nagurney, J.   Progressive supranuclear opthalmoplegia. *Journal of the American Medical Association,* 1977, *237,* 994–995.

Siegel, C., Hendrix, T., & Collins, J.   The swallowing disorder in myotonia dystrophica. *Gastroenterology,* 1966, *50,* 541–549.

Silbiger, M., Pikielney, R., & Donner, M.   Neuromuscular disorders affecting the pharynx: Cineradiographic analysis. *Investigative Radiology,* 1967, *2,* 442–448.

Sloan, R.   The cinefluorographic study of cerebral palsy deglutition patterns. *Journal of Osaka Dental University,* 1977, *11,* 58–73.

Smith, A., Mulder, D., & Code, C.   Esophageal motility in amyotrophic lateral sclerosis. *Mayo Clinic Proceedings of the Staff Meetings,* 1957, *32,* 438–441.

Sparberg, M., Knudsen, K., & Frank, S.   Dysautonomia and dysphagia. *Neurology,* 1968, *18,* 504–506.

Walker, J., Singer, K., & Baker, P.   Disorders of esophageal motility in a family with hereditary spastic ataxia. *Neurology,* 1969, *19,* 1212–1216.

9

Medical Treatment for Swallowing Disorders

Techniques Designed to Improve Specific Swallowing Disorders

There are several medical procedures designed to improve specific types of swallowing disorders. These include surgical reduction of osteophytes, teflon injection into the reconstructed or damaged vocal fold to improve vocal fold closure and airway protection during swallowing, and dilatation or cricopharyngeal myotomy to open the sphincter at the top of the esophagus.

Surgical Reduction of Osteophytes

Cervical osteophytes are boney overgrowths on the cervical vertebra that displace the posterior pharyngeal wall anteriorly. If the pharyngeal narrowing is severe, surgical reduction can be performed by entering the paraesophageal space through an incision in the side of the neck (Blumberg, Prapote, & Viscomi, 1977). The vertebral periosteum is reflected back and the excess bone removed. There is some difference of opinion on the effect of cervical osteophytes on swallowing. There is no doubt that if a cervical osteophyte is large enough, the mass of bone can significantly diminish the pharyngeal space, making the passage of a large or thick bolus of food difficult. Or, as Press and Leffall (1972) report, the boney overgrowth may press on the cervical nerve roots, producing the sense of dysphagia.

Teflon Injection into
the Reconstructed or
Damaged Vocal Fold

Teflon injection into the vocal cord is a procedure that adds bulk to one vocal cord or to whatever tissue is located at the top of the airway in order to improve closure and airway protection during swallowing. The additional mass of teflon is added to the damaged or reconstructed vocal fold and is thought to improve contact with the other, movable vocal fold, thus, facilitating closure (Arnold, 1962; Lewy, 1963; Sessions, Zill, & Schwartz, 1979). The technique is frequently used in patients whose laryngeal adduction for airway protection cannot be improved with an exercise program. It has been used in head and neck surgical patients, particularly partial laryngectomy patients whose remaining tissues in the larynx are insufficient to adduct and protect the airway. One limitation to the procedure is the denseness of the tissue into which the injection is made. There must be enough tissue space to accept the teflon. Teflon has also been used in neurologic patients with inadequate vocal fold closure, including individuals with Parkinson's disease and amyotrophic lateral sclerosis (ALS). If the swallowing disorder causing aspiration is, in fact, reduced laryngeal closure, teflon injection may be a successful treatment. If, however, the procedure is done on patients whose swallowing has not been carefully evaluated radiographically, and who are aspirating because of reduced lingual control, delayed or absent reflex, or reduced pharyngeal peristalsis, adding teflon to the adductor mechanism will not improve the swallow or reduce the aspiration. Often, before injecting teflon, glycerine or some other *temporary* substance is injected to simulate the effect of the teflon. The glycerine will be absorbed into the tissues and will disappear in approximately a week. In the interim, the patient's changed function as a result of the increased mass created by the glycerine can be assessed, and the importance of performing the injection with teflon can be determined.

Dilatation of
the Cricopharyngeus
Sphincter

Dilatation of the cricopharyngeus involves the passage of mercury-filled soft rubber tubes (bougies) of increasing diameter through the cricopharyngeus to gradually stretch it open. Most clinicians have found the effects of the dilatation to be temporary, lasting approximately 1 month (Calcaterra, Kadell, & Ward, 1975; Palmer, 1974). Because of the increased resistance at the upper esophageal sphincter in these patients, it may be difficult to pass the bougie through the muscle, and a perforation can occur (Duranceau et al. 1978).

Cricopharyngeal Myotomy

Cricopharyngeal myotomy has been used to treat swallowing disorders in a number of patients, including those with Parkinson's disease, ALS, and occulopharyngeal dystrophy (Aki & Blakely, 1974; Asherson, 1973; Calcaterra et al., 1975; Dayal & Freeman, 1976; Duranceau et al., 1978; Ellis, Schlegel, Lynch & Payne, 1969; Henderson & Marryatt, 1977; Mills, 1964; Palmer, 1974; Stevens & Newell, 1971; Wilkins, 1964). The procedure involves an external incision through the side of the neck (usually the left side) into the cricopharyngeal muscle, slitting the muscle from top to bottom, usually at the posterior midline, to permanently open the sphincter. Usually the incision extends upward to include the inferior constrictor fibers, and downward into the esophageal musculature (Calcaterra et al., 1975). The patient frequently can begin to eat within 1 week after the myotomy (Mitchell & Armanini, 1975). Studies of the success of this procedure have sometimes reported improvement rates of 60 to 78% (Lebo, Sang U, & Norris, 1976; Mills, 1973). When the criteria used for selection of patients in these studies are carefully examined, it is often clear that patients with swallowing disorders other than cricopharyngeal dysfunction have been treated with this surgery. The success of the myotomy in those patients would be negligible and thus affect the success rate of the procedure. Success rates for myotomy climb when patients are carefully selected for the procedure using the following criteria: (1) the cricopharyngeal dysfunction must be the predominant problem; (2) the patient must be able to move material through the oral and pharyngeal stages of the swallow up to the cricopharyngeus; and (3) the patient must be able to voluntarily close the airway during the swallow (Aki & Blakeley, 1974; Blakeley, Garety, & Smith, 1968; Wilkins, 1964).

Some patients who have received a myotomy may not benefit from it unless a postural assist is also used. The patient is usually asked to turn his or her head toward the unoperated side, thus directing material through the pyriform sinus on the operated, and presumably the more open, side. Patients with multiple dysfunctions in the vocal tract including reduced lingual control, delayed swallowing reflex, or reduced pharyngeal peristalsis, in addition to cricopharyngeal dysfunction, are generally poor candidates for the procedure since the myotomy will only open the sphincter at the bottom of the pharynx. It will not improve transit to that point. If the swallowing reflex does not trigger, the larynx will stand open to receive any material that drains over the base of the tongue into the pharynx. Even with a relaxed cricopharyngeus, material is just as likely to drain into the open airway as it is to drain into the open esophagus. Complications of the procedure may include hemorrhage or recurrent laryngeal nerve damage, as well as complications inherent in opening the pharynx or esophagus (Lund, 1968).

Techniques for Non-Oral Feeding

Several procedures can be used to feed patients who are unable to take nutrition by mouth. These include nasogastric feeding or the variants, pharyngostomy or esophagostomy, and gastrostomy, or jejunostomy.

Nasogastric Feeding (NG Tube)

This technique utilizes a tube placed through the nose, pharynx, and esophagus into the stomach. The diameter of the tubes vary; however, a narrow tube is preferred to create minimal irritation in the pharynx. particularly as the tube passes through the cricopharyngeal juncture at the top of the esophagus. Food is passed through the tube into the stomach. The number of feedings per day and amount of food given per feeding vary from one hospital to another. However, each feeding is usually followed by at least 120 to 240cc of water to cleanse the feeding tube and provide proper hydration (Sessions et al., 1979).

Disadvantages of the nasogastric tube are its physical presence in the pharynx and esophagus and the potential for regurgitation of food up the esophagus into the pharynx. Also, the feeding usually consists of prepared liquid diets that can be expensive.

The Dophoff tube is designed to reduce the potential for reflux and aspiration by extending into the jejunum. It is of a small diameter and, presumably, creates less irritation in the pharynx.

Nasogastric feeding is generally considered a temporary solution to problems with oral feeding, and is usually replaced with a more permanent procedure after 3 to 4 months. However, some types of patients may have a nasogastric tube in place for 5 or 6 months, or longer. These patients can be taught to place the nasogastric tube themselves so it can be put in for each meal and removed after feeding.

Pharyngostomy

A pharyngostomy involves creation of a hole or stoma from the skin into the pharynx through which a tube is placed into the esophagus and, thence, the stomach. The advantages of the pharyngostomy over the nasogastric tube is the elimination of the tube through the nose, which is irritating to many patients. Its disadvantage is the creation of a hole that may need to be closed surgically. Some head and neck cancer patients develop a pharyngostomy spontaneously.

Esophagostomy

An esophagostomy is a hole from the skin into the cervical esophagus through which a feeding tube is passed which extends into the esophagus and stomach. Its advantages and disadvantages are similar to those of the pharyngostomy.

Gastrostomy

The gastrostomy is a surgical procedure that creates an external opening in the abdomen leading into the stomach. The patient wears a light dressing on the opening, designed to close in sphinctric fashion around a soft tube. For feeding, food is passed through the tube directly into the stomach. The patient can take blenderized table food through the tube.

The procedure is generally considered a long-term solution to a severe swallowing disorder because it removes the risk of nasal and pharyngeal irritation from a nasogastric tube. It can be reversed should the patient regain the ability to eat by mouth. Its disadvantage is that the stoma site can leak, or can become infected or sore and uncomfortable.

Criteria for Implementation of a Non-Oral Feeding Procedure

Use of a non-oral feeding procedure should stabilize a patient's nutritional needs. Any patient who is aspirating significantly (more than 10% of all food consistencies) or who is taking longer than 10 seconds to swallow a single bolus of food, regardless of consistency, is a candidate for a non-oral feeding technique to at least supplement nutritional intake. In general, if the patient's swallowing disorder is thought to be short-term in nature (3 months or less), a nasogastric tube is the treatment of choice. If swallowing rehabilitation is anticipated to take more than 3 months, a gastrostomy may be more appropriate, unless the patient can be taught to place the nasogastric tube for each meal, and remove it between meals.

Bibliography

Aki, B., & Blakeley, W.   Late assessment of results of cricopharyngeal myotomy for cervical dysphagia. *American Journal of Surgery,* 1974, *128,* 818–821.

Arnold G.   Vocal rehabilitation of paralytic dysphonia: IX technique of intracordal injection. *Archives of Otolaryngology,* 1962, *76,* 358–368.

Asherson, N.   Dysphagia in pharyngeal paralysis treated by cricopharyngeal sphincterotomy. *Lancet,* 1973, *1,* 722.

Blakeley, W., Garety, E., & Smith, D.   Section of the cricopharyngeus muscle for dysphagia. *Archives of Surgery,* 1968, *96,* 745–762.

Blumberg, D., Prapote, C., & Viscomi, G.   Cervical osteophytes producing dysphagia. *Ear, Nose and Throat Journal,* 1977, *56,* 15–21.

Calcaterra, T., Kadell, B., & Ward, P.   Dysphagia secondary to cricopharyngeal muscle dysfunction. *Archives of Otolaryngology,* 1975, *101,* 726–729.

Chodosh, P.   Cricopharyngeal myotomy in the treatment of dysphagia. *Laryngoscope,* 1975, *85,* 1862–1873.

Cruse, J., Edwards, D., Smith, J., & Wyllie, J.   The pathology of a cricopharyngeal dysphagia. *Histopathology,* 1979, *3,* 223–232.

Dayal, T., & Freeman, J.   Cricopharyngeal myotomy for dysphagia in oculopharyngeal muscular dystrophy. *Archives of Otolaryngology,* 1976, *102,* 115–116.

Duranceau, C., Letendre, J., Clermont, R., Levesque, H., & Barbeau, A.   Oropharyngeal dysphagia in patients with oculopharyngeal muscular dystrophy. *The Canadian Journal of Surgery,* 1978, *21,* 326–329.

Ellis, F., Schlegel, J., Lynch, V., & Payne, W.   Cricopharyngeal myotomy for pharyngoesophageal diverticulum. *Annals of Surgery,* 1969, *170,* 340–350.

Henderson, R., & Marryatt, G.   Cricopharyngeal myotomy as a method of treating cricopharyngeal dysphagia secondary to gastroesophageal reflux. *Journal of Thoracic and Cardiovascular Surgery,* 1977, *74,* 721–725.

Lebo, C., Sang U, K., & Norris, F.   Cricopharyngeal myotomy in amyotrophic lateral sclerosis. *Laryngoscope, 1976, 86,* 862–868.

Lewy, R.,   Glottic reformation with voice rehabilitation in vocal cord paralysis. *Laryngoscope,* 1963, *73,* 547–555.

Lund, W.   The cricopharyngeal sphincter: Its relationship to the relief of pharyngeal paralysis and the surgical treatment of the early pharyngeal pouch. *Journal of Laryngology and Otology,* 1968, *82,* 353–367.

Mills, C.   Dysphagia in progressive bulbar palsy relieved by division of the cricopharyngeus. *Journal of Laryngology and Otology,* 1964, *78,* 963–964.

Mills, C.   Dysphagia in pharyngeal paralysis treated by cricopharyngeal sphincterotomy. *Lancet,* 1973, *1,* 455–457.

Mitchell, R., & Armanini, G.   Cricopharyngeal myotomy: Treatment of dysphagia. *Annals of Surgery,* 1975, *181,* 262–266.

Mladick, R., Horton, C., & Adamson, J.   Cricopharyngeal myotomy. *Archives of Surgery,* 1971, *102* (6), 1–5.

Mladick, R., Horton, C., & Adamson, J.   Immediate cricopharyngeal myotomy: An adjunctive technique for major oral-pharyngeal resections. *Plastic and Reconstructive Surgery,* 1961, *47,* 6–11.

Palmer, E.   Dysphagia due to cricopharyngeus dysfunction. *American Family Physician,* 1974, *9,* 127–131.

Press, H., & Leffall, L.   Hoarseness and dysphagia secondary to cervical hyperostosis: Report of an unusual case. *Medical Annals of the District of Columbia,* 1972, *41,* 26–28.

Sessions, D., Zill, R., & Schwartz, J.   Deglutition after conservation surgery for cancer of the larynx and hypopharynx. *Otolaryngology, Head and Neck Surgery,* 1979, *87,* 779–796.

Stevens, K., & Newell, R.   Cricopharyngeal myotomy in dysphagia. *Laryngoscope,* 1971, *81,* 1616–1620.

Wilkins, S   Indications for section of the cricopharyngeus muscle. *American Journal of Surgery,* 1964, *108,* 533–538.

Yarington, C., & Harned, R.   Polytef (teflon) injection for postoperative deglutition problems. *Archives of Otolaryngology,* 1971, *94,* 274–275.

Zinninger, G.   Dysphagia & esophageal dilatation. *Journal of the American Medical Association,* 1966, *196,* 128–129.

Author Index

Subject Index

Bold type numbers denote material in table or figure.